The Secret B[...]f relationsnips, love and sex™

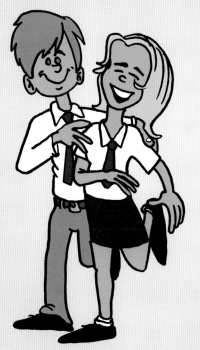

Written by
Heather Anderson
Fay Angelo
Rose Stewart
Illustrated by
Jeff Taylor

This is a young persons' guide to friendships, relationships, love and sex.

It provides information about the physical changes associated with puberty, changing relationships, love, sex and staying safe.

SGB Publishing

CONTENTS

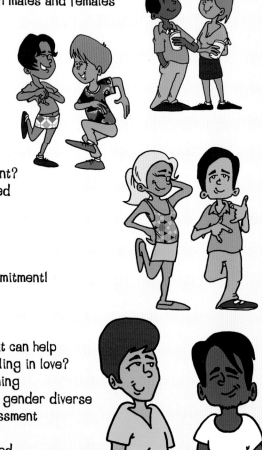

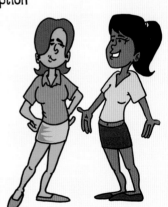

People grow and change

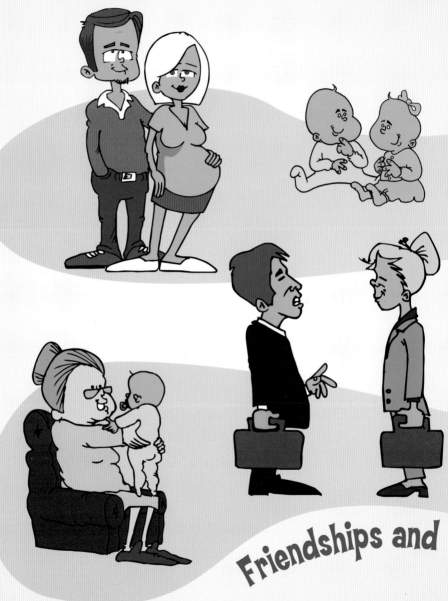

Friendships and

all through their lives

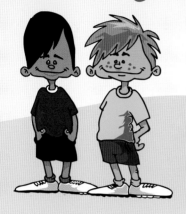

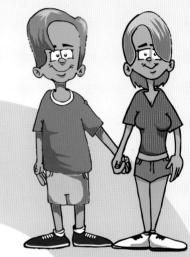

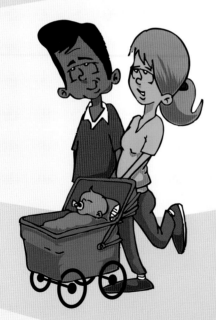

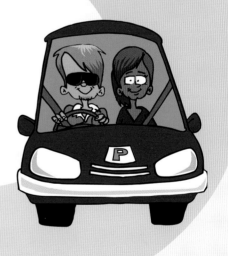

relationships change also

Puberty

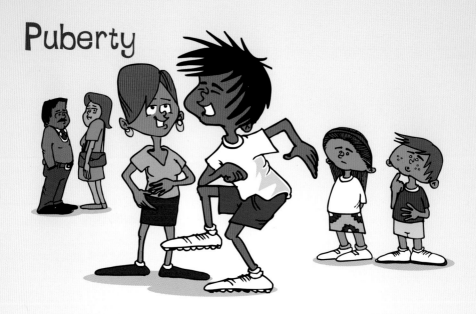

At puberty, there are changes in the way bodies look and work and also the way young people think and feel. More hormones are produced at this time. Hormones contain chemical messages which are carried in the blood, causing:

- The body to gradually change from a child to an adult.
- Emotional changes such as mood variations and sexy thoughts and feelings.

The most important male hormone is testosterone, which is produced in the testicles.

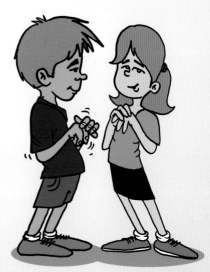

The most important female hormones are oestrogen and progesterone. They are produced in the ovaries.

Puberty begins at different ages in different people.

Girls usually begin puberty between 8 and 16 years old.

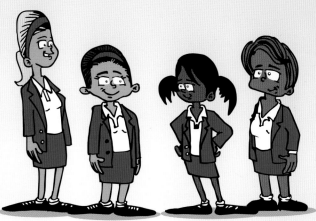

Puberty in boys usually begins between 9 and 17 years of age.

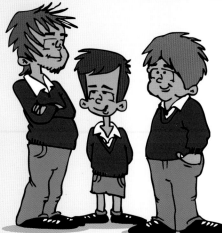

This means that some girls will be taller and more physically developed than boys of the same age for a year or two, until boys have their growth spurt.

If young people are worried about any aspects of puberty, they can talk to a trusted adult or a doctor.

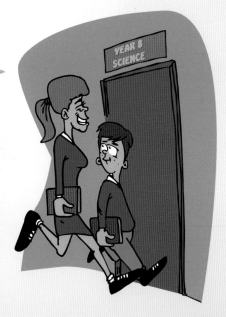

YEAR 8
SCIENCE

Puberty changes to

- A noticeable growth spurt.
- Muscles develop, bodies become stronger.
- The brain develops. Young people are smarter and more capable of logical reasoning
- They become more responsible and independent.

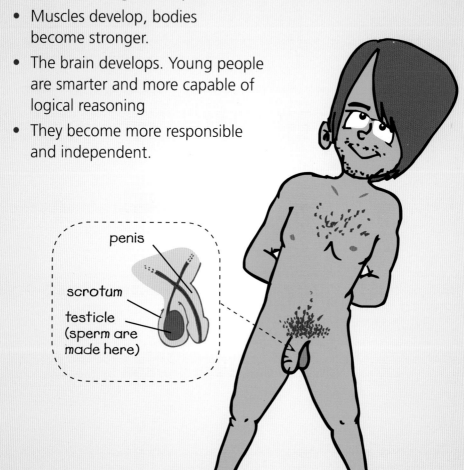

penis

scrotum

testicle
(sperm are
made here)

both males and females

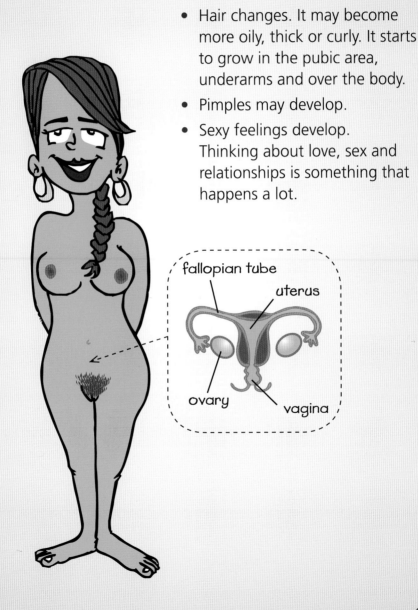

- Hair changes. It may become more oily, thick or curly. It starts to grow in the pubic area, underarms and over the body.
- Pimples may develop.
- Sexy feelings develop. Thinking about love, sex and relationships is something that happens a lot.

fallopian tube

uterus

ovary

vagina

MALE CHANGES

At puberty the testicles increase testosterone production, which brings about characteristic male changes:

- Hair grows on the face.
- Voice changes and deepens, caused by rapid growth in the larynx (voice box) and vocal chords.
- Changes to the genitals – the penis and testicles.

Inside the jocks

For boys some of the most significant puberty changes happen inside their jocks.

The penis and testicles develop and enlarge. The testicles hang lower and the scrotum becomes darker in colour. Pubic hair grows around the base of the penis, over the scrotum and around the anus.

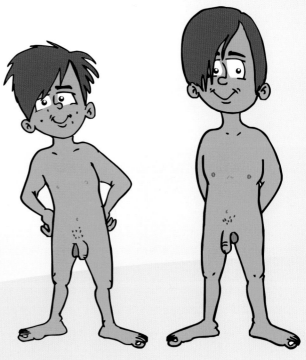

Penises vary in shape, size and colour. This is normal. Whatever shape or size, the penis performs the same functions: urinating, ejaculating semen and bringing sexual pleasure.

The penis has many nerve endings that make it sensitive. The tip or head of the penis is the most sensitive part. The long part of the penis is called the shaft.

When a boy is born the tip of the penis is covered by a foreskin. Some boys have surgery to remove the foreskin. This small operation, called circumcision, leaves the head of the penis visible.

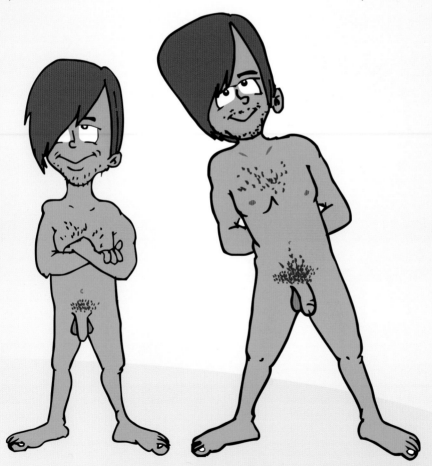

Erections

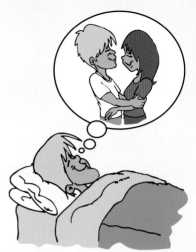

The penis becomes erect when extra blood flows into it, causing it to become bigger, straighter and stiff.

Erections occur in response to sexy thoughts, stimulation (rubbing or touching) of the penis, and sometimes for no reason at all.

At puberty, while physical changes are happening, there are also changes in thoughts and feelings. Lots of boys will be thinking about love and sex. Boys may have frequent erections, which may be embarrassing.

Unwanted erections will disappear more quickly if boys try to concentrate or focus on something else. Erections are less noticeable if loose clothing is worn.

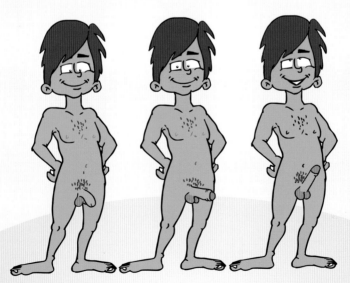

Sperm production

At puberty the increase in testosterone triggers the testicles to produce sperm, and semen which nourishes and protects the sperm. Up to 1 billion sperm are produced each day. Sperm are so small they can only be seen through a microscope.

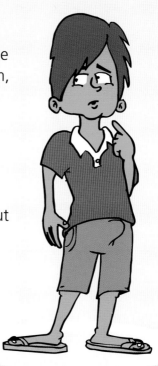

Males may have frequent erections but usually only ejaculate (release sperm and semen from the penis) during masturbation, a wet dream or sexual intercourse.

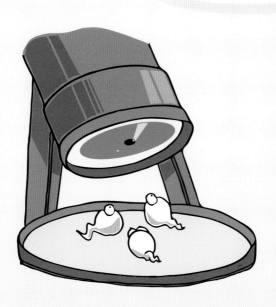

Wet dreams

When a male is having a sexy or exciting dream he may ejaculate sperm and semen. This is called a 'wet dream'. He may wake during ejaculation with a very enjoyable feeling called an orgasm.

An orgasm is a very strong, pleasurable feeling in the genital area that lasts for a short time. This is followed by a feeling of warmth, wellbeing and relaxation.

The number of wet dreams experienced can vary greatly from boy to boy.

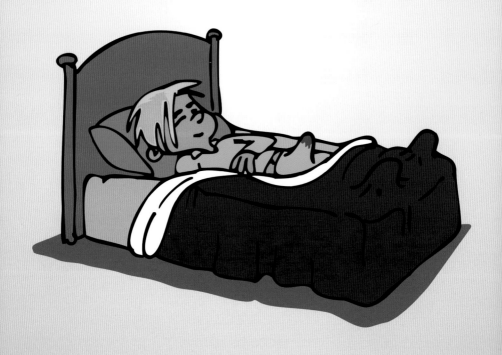

Masturbation

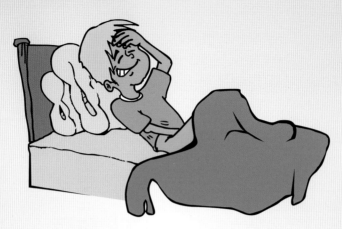

At puberty it is normal for boys to often think about love, sex and relationships. They may have tingly and enjoyable feelings in the body and penis. Some males choose to masturbate in private when they have these feelings.

Masturbation is rubbing the penis, which brings about exciting and intense enjoyable feelings leading to orgasm and ejaculation.

Masturbation is normal. Most boys masturbate, some often and some occasionally.

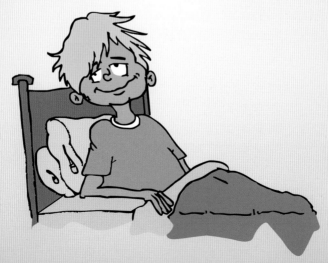

FeMALe CHANGeS

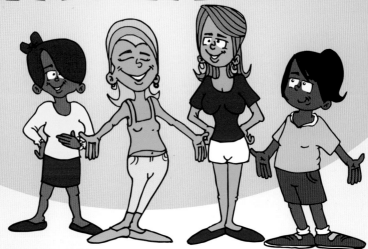

At puberty the ovaries begin to produce more oestrogen and progesterone, which brings about characteristic female changes:

- breast development,
- widening of the hips,
- growth and development of the vagina and reproductive organs, and
- periods begin.

Curvy bits

Breasts

A significant female body change that occurs at puberty is the growth of breasts.

Breast development begins with a breast bud: a small lump that can be felt behind the nipple. Nipples gradually become bigger and the areola, the skin around the nipples, becomes darker.

It is common for girls (and boys) to have flat or turned in (inverted) nipples. Some girls will notice a few hairs growing around the nipple. This is normal.

Often one breast is a little bigger than the other.

At puberty breasts can be tender, itchy or sensitive.

Breasts vary greatly in shape and size. Size does not affect the ability to feed a baby after birth.

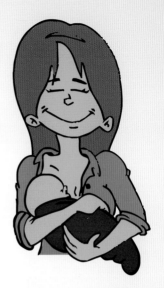

Hips

At puberty the bony pelvic opening widens to allow for the birth of a baby in the future. This changes the body shape, widening the hips and accentuating the waist.

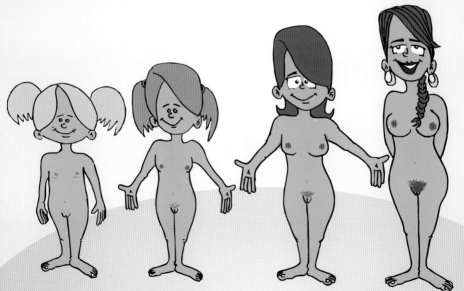

Changes down below

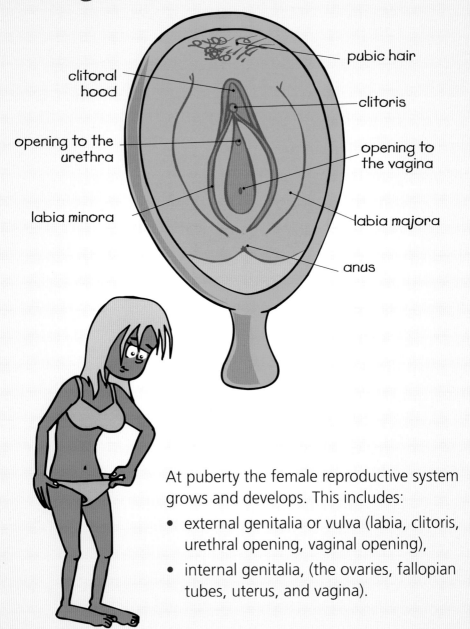

pubic hair

clitoral hood

clitoris

opening to the urethra

opening to the vagina

labia minora

labia majora

anus

At puberty the female reproductive system grows and develops. This includes:

- external genitalia or vulva (labia, clitoris, urethral opening, vaginal opening),
- internal genitalia, (the ovaries, fallopian tubes, uterus, and vagina).

Vaginal discharge

At puberty girls will notice a very small amount of discharge that comes out of the vagina each day and can be seen in the undies. It keeps the vagina moist. Vaginal discharge can vary in thickness and colour during the menstrual cycle, from clear to white or cream. This is normal and healthy. The appearance of vaginal discharge is a sign that periods will begin in the next 6–12 months.

At times, some girls may develop an infection in the genital area, which can be easily treated.

Seek medical advice if:

- Vaginal discharge changes from the normal colour or has an offensive smell.
- The vagina or vulva is itchy or sore.
- Urination (having a wee) is painful.

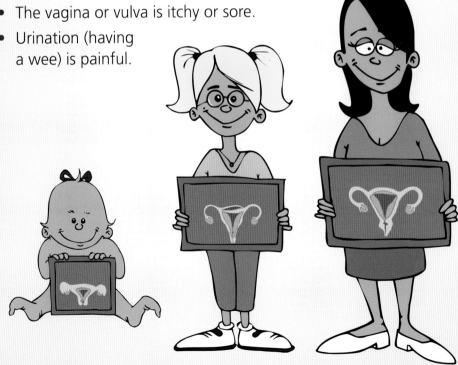

Periods

A period is a small amount of blood (about 2–3 tablespoons) which comes slowly out of the vagina each month. Pads or tampons are worn to absorb this blood.

The uterus forms a lining of blood to nourish a developing baby. If a baby is not conceived, the uterus sheds the lining and the blood dribbles slowly out of the vagina. This is called a 'period'.

Menstrual cycle

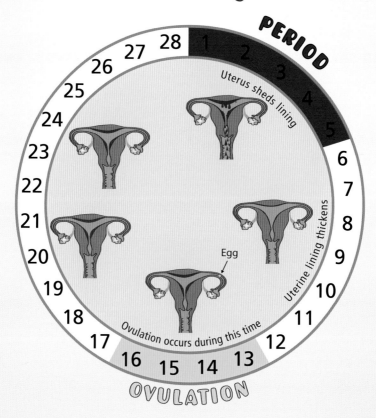

Uterus sheds lining

Uterine lining thickens

Egg

Ovulation occurs during this time

PERIOD

OVULATION

As soon as the period is finished, a new lining begins to form. An ovum (egg) will mature and be released from the ovary (ovulation) approximately 2 weeks before the next period. If the ovum is not fertilized by a sperm, the lining of blood in the uterus comes away and leaves the body as the next period.

This series of changes is called the 'menstrual cycle'.

The menstrual cycle continues until women reach menopause at about the age of 50.

S	M	T	W	T	F	S
				1	2	3
4	5	6	7	8	9	10
11	12	13	14	15	16	17
18	19	20	21	22	23	24
25	26	27	28	29	30	

When periods first happen, the time between them can vary greatly. After several cycles however, periods become more regular and usually occur each month, lasting 3–7 days. The blood flow may be light, moderate or heavier.

MARCH						
S	M	T	W	T	F	S
				1	2	3
4	5	6	7	8	9	10
11	12	13	14	15	16	17
18	19	20	21	22	23	24
25	26	27	28	29	30	31

APRIL						
S	M	T	W	T	F	S
1	2	3	4	5	6	7
8	9	10	11	12	13	14
15	16	17	18	19	20	21
22	23	24	25	26	27	28
29	30					

MAY						
S	M	T	W	T	F	S
		1	2	3	4	5
6	7	8	9	10	11	12
13	14	15	16	17	18	19
20	21	22	23	24	25	26
27	28	29	30	31		

JUNE						
S	M	T	W	T	F	S
					1	2
3	4	5	6	7	8	9
10	11	12	13	14	15	16
17	18	19	20	21	22	23
24	25	26	27	28	29	30

JULY						
S	M	T	W	T	F	S
1	2	3	4	5	6	7
8	9	10	11	12	13	14
15	16	17	18	19	20	21
22	23	24	25	26	27	28
29	30	31				

AUGUST						
S	M	T	W	T	F	S
			1	2	3	4
5	6	7	8	9	10	11
12	13	14	15	16	17	18
19	20	21	22	23	24	25
26	27	28	29	30	31	

SEPTEMBER						
S	M	T	W	T	F	S
						1
2	3	4	5	6	7	8
9	10	11	12	13	14	15
16	17	18	19	20	21	22
23	24	25	26	27	28	29
30						

Many girls will experience some discomfort in the lower abdomen during a period. Some girls find heat packs or medication helpful.

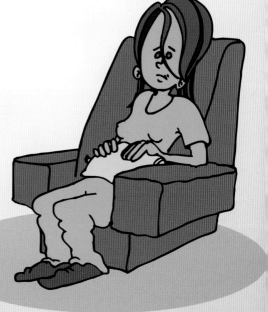

Exercise and relaxing activities can help too.

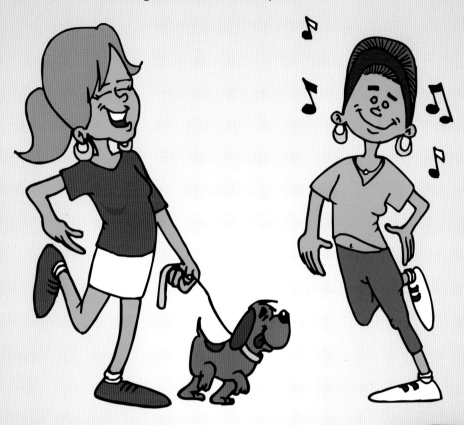

Some girls may experience pre-menstrual syndrome (PMS) in the time leading up to their period. They may be teary, irritable, have tender breasts, pimples or discomfort in the abdomen.

If there are concerns about anything to do with periods talk to a doctor.

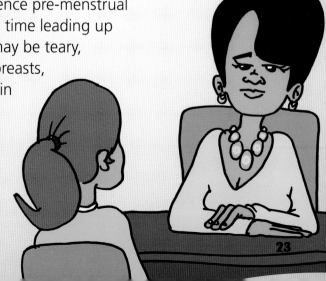

Private moments

At puberty it is normal for girls to think about love, sex and relationships. The body produces more female hormones that cause an increase in sexy feelings. These are warm, tingly feelings in the nipples, vulva and vagina. Nipples are extra-sensitive and respond to touch, temperature and sexual thoughts and feelings by becoming harder and erect. When females have sexy thoughts their vagina and vulva may become moist. Some girls may choose to masturbate when they have sexy feelings.

Masturbation is touching or rubbing the clitoris and vulva. This may give very pleasant enjoyable feelings. If stimulation of the clitoris and vulva continues, an orgasm may occur.

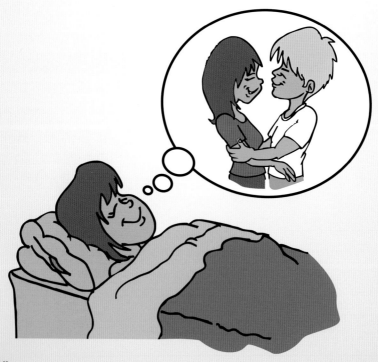

An orgasm is an intense pleasurable feeling around the genital area that is a very strong for a moment. It fades and is followed by a feeling of warmth, wellbeing and relaxation.

Masturbation is a way for girls and young women to discover how their body feels and works. This is part of normal development.

Many girls will masturbate. Some girls will not feel comfortable exploring their body in this way.

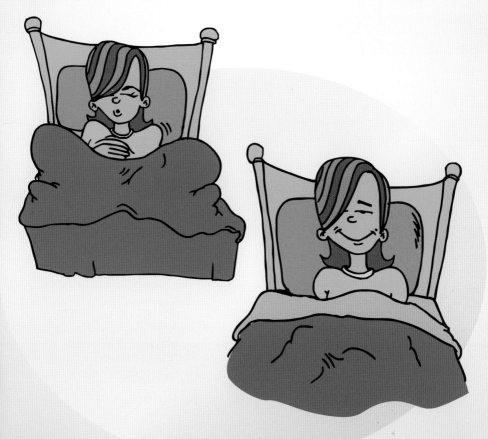

PUBERTY! - WHAT'S

At puberty, the female reproductive system develops and ovulation begins. In males, sperm production commences.
These changes make it possible for a baby to be conceived.

This is nature's way of ensuring that the human race continues.

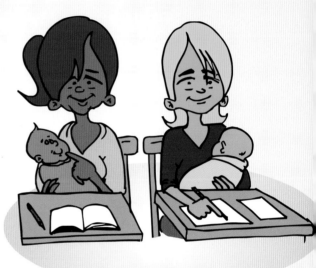

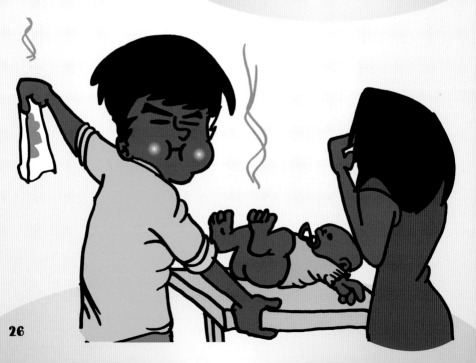

THE POINT?

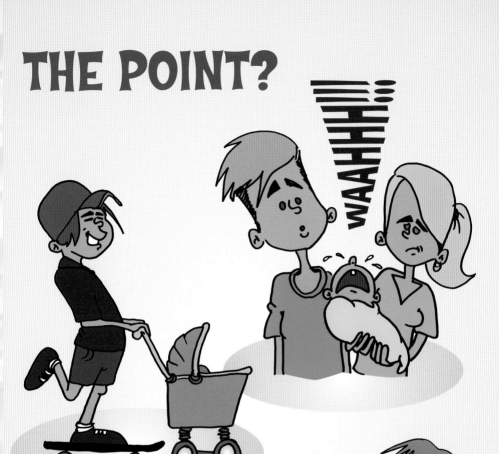

Although a boy and a girl may be physically able to create a baby when they are about 12 years old, most young people would not be emotionally ready or financially capable of coping with the challenges of raising a child.

How babies are conceived

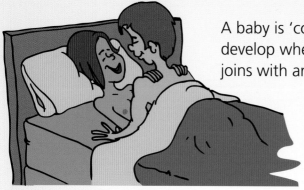

A baby is 'conceived' or starts to develop when sperm from a male joins with an egg from a female.

This usually happens as a result of sexual intercourse when a male's penis is in a female's vagina. Their bodies move together and after a short time the male ejaculates into the vagina. The sperm travels up the vagina, through the uterus and into the fallopian tubes. If the sperm joins with an egg, a baby begins to form.

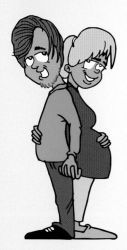

Babies made in different ways

Not all babies are conceived as a result of sexual intercourse.

Babies may also be created by:

IVF (In Vitro Fertilization)

A medical procedure during which eggs are taken from the ovaries and placed in a container with sperm. When an egg has been fertilized, the embryo is surgically inserted into the uterus. Couples may choose IVF if they have difficulty getting pregnant.

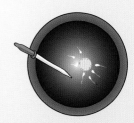

⚥ Donor sperm

Donated sperm is collected and stored in a medical facility. The semen is inserted into the woman's vagina. If a sperm joins with an egg, a baby is conceived.

⚥ Donor eggs

The egg is collected from another woman during a small operation. This donated egg is fertilized by IVF with the father's sperm, then placed in the mother's uterus.

⚥ Surrogacy

When a woman is pregnant and gives birth on behalf of another couple.

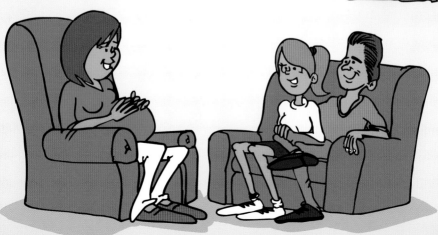

The developing baby

After fertilization, the new cell multiplies forming a tiny ball of cells. The ball of cells moves down the fallopian tube to the uterus where it attaches to the nutritious lining.

A number of important changes immediately begin to take place:

- The placenta forms. The placenta connects the embryo to the mother's blood supply.

- The umbilical cord forms. This cord contains blood vessels that transport nutrition and oxygen from the placenta to the developing baby, and carry waste products from the baby's blood back to the placenta and to the mother's blood stream.

- The amniotic sac forms around the embryo. It is like a small balloon filled with amniotic fluid. It supports and protects the developing baby.

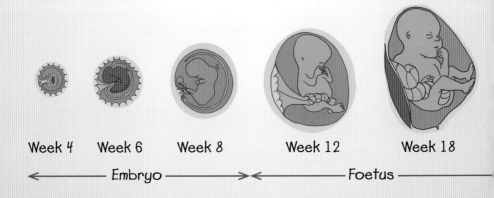

Week 4   Week 6   Week 8   Week 12   Week 18

⟵——————— Embryo ———————⟶⟵——————— Foetus ———————

The developing baby is called an embryo at four weeks, then after 10 weeks of the pregnancy it is called a foetus.

The foetus grows and develops in the uterus for about 9 months. Then it is ready to be born.

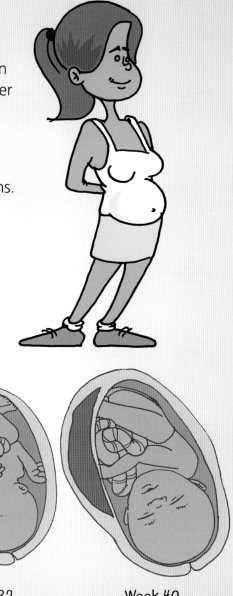

Week 24   Week 32   Week 40

The birth process

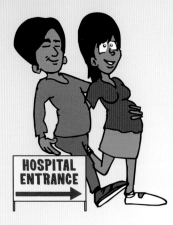

The birth date is calculated by counting on 40 weeks from the first day of the mother's last period before conception.

The process of the baby leaving the mother's body is called 'labour'.

Labour starts when the strong muscles of the uterus begin to squeeze and relax. This is called a 'contraction'. With each contraction the mother feels a strong ache or pain across her lower abdomen. The contractions gradually become more frequent, get stronger and last longer. The cervix gradually stretches, becomes thinner, and forms an opening about 10 cm in diameter. The mother now feels a very strong urge to push with each contraction. This moves the baby out of the uterus, through the vagina, and it is born!

Most babies are born head first but some may be born feet or bottom first (breach birth).

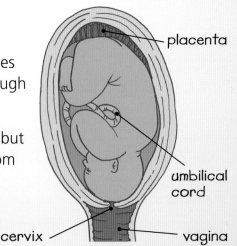

placenta

umbilical cord

cervix

vagina

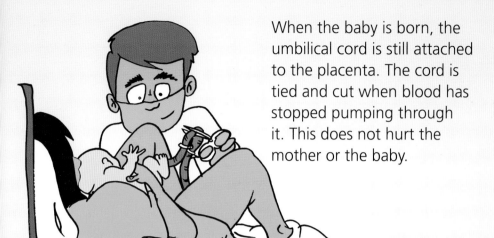

When the baby is born, the umbilical cord is still attached to the placenta. The cord is tied and cut when blood has stopped pumping through it. This does not hurt the mother or the baby.

Once the cord is cut, the baby is no longer receiving oxygen from the mother so it will now have to start breathing independently.

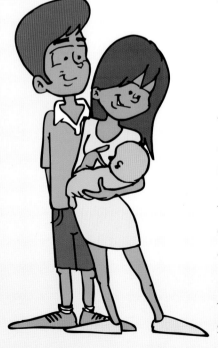

The final stage of labour happens after the baby is born. The placenta detaches from the uterus and comes easily out of the vagina with the umbilical cord and the placental sac attached.

Most babies will start to learn to suck on their mother's breast soon after birth.

Caesarean birth

Not all babies are born through the vagina. Some are born by 'Caesarean section', a surgical procedure used to deliver a baby.

Before a caesarean birth, the mother has an anaesthetic so that she does not feel any pain. The doctor then carefully cuts an opening (incision) in the lower abdomen through to the uterus and lifts the baby out, then the placenta.

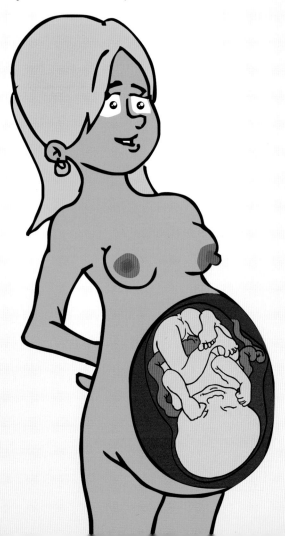

The cord is tied and cut. The incision is then carefully stitched together again. A baby might be born by Caesarean because:

- It is not in the 'head down' position.
- The baby's health is at risk.
- The baby is not moving down the birth canal despite ongoing contractions.
- The mother chooses a caesarian birth.

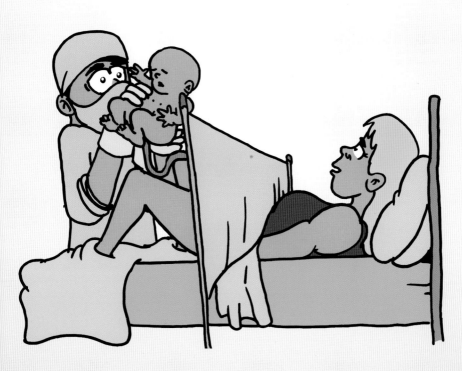

How many babies?

A single birth occurs when one egg (ovum) is fertilized by one sperm.

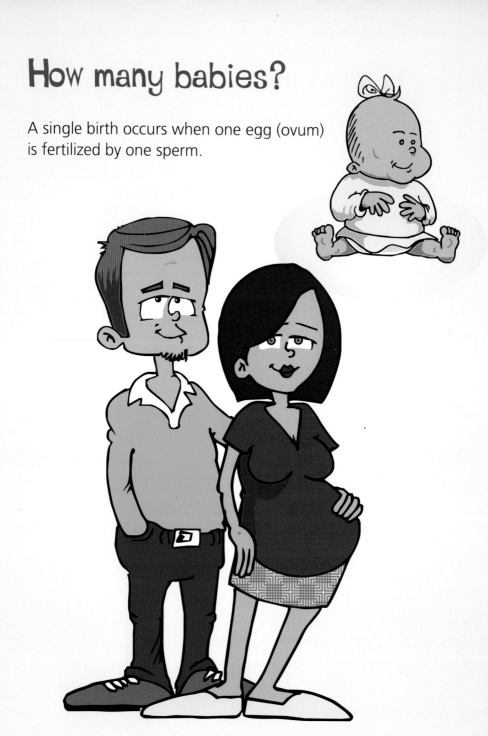

Identical multiple births

Identical twins, triplets, quadruplets are formed when one ovum is fertilized by one sperm and then divides into two (forming twins), three (forming triplets) or four (quadruplets or 'quads')

Non-identical multiple births

Non identical twins, triplets and quads are formed when two or more eggs are released from the ovaries at the same time and each egg is separately fertilized by a different sperm.

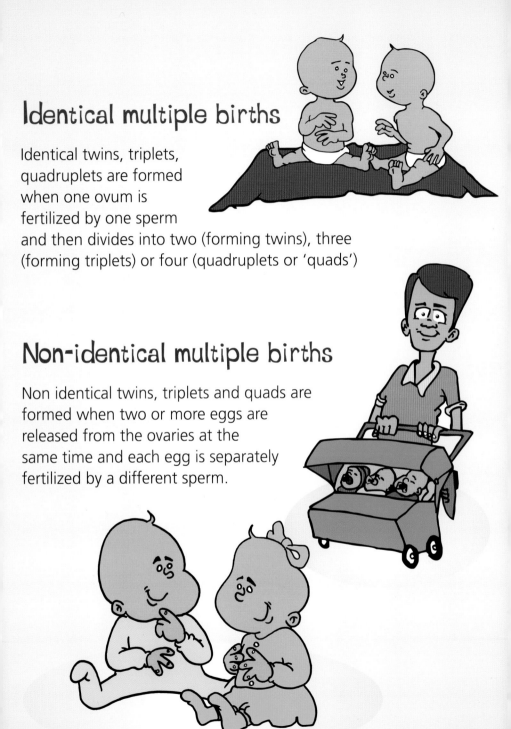

PARENTING

To bring a 'new life' into the world is usually a joyous occasion for both parents. However, this may not be the case if a pregnancy is unplanned.

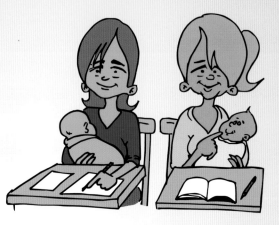

Looking after a baby is an important responsibility for parents and is not always easy. New babies need to be looked after very carefully, all day and also at night. The parents are often woken up and may become exhausted.

Babies need food, shelter, nappies, clean clothes, pusher, pram, cot, baby bath, toys, car seat, books, visits to the doctor, medicine and many other things! Having a baby is expensive!

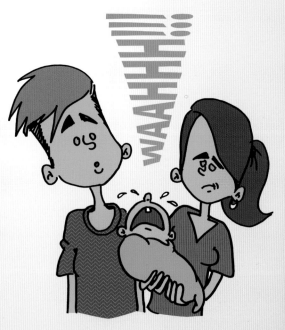

A huge commitment!

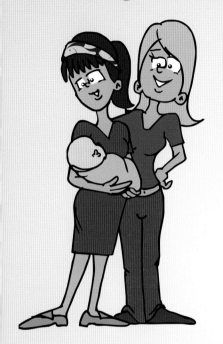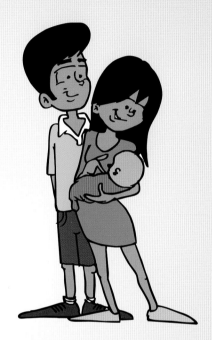

Most importantly however, babies need constant attention and love. All babies and children have the right to lots of love, care, and protection.

It is good to wait, think ahead, plan carefully and choose the right time – when the parents are both ready, and capable of looking after and caring for their baby. This will mean that the birth of a baby is a joyous occasion!

Relationships

At puberty, our bodies gradually change, and so do our thoughts and feelings, and the way we interact with others. Our friendships and relationships gradually change as we mature.

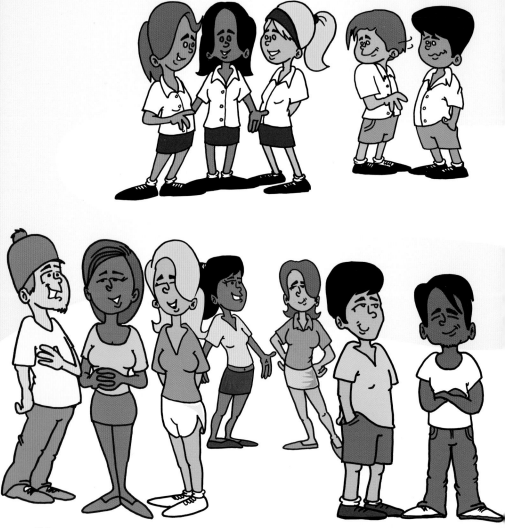

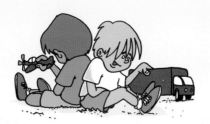

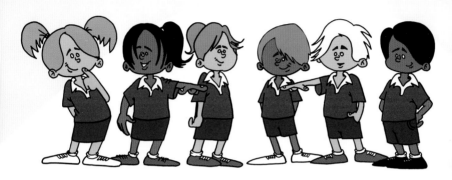

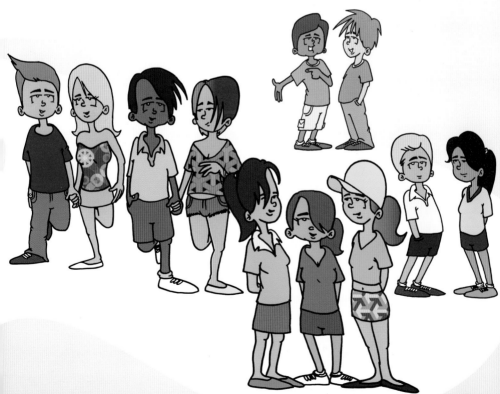

Friendships

During the teen years it is usual to have some old friends and some new friends, and to move in and out of friendship groups. It can be good to have two or three friends because people who spend all their time with one friend can feel lonely if that friend is not around. Getting to know different people helps us learn how to understand and get along with others and makes our lives more interesting.

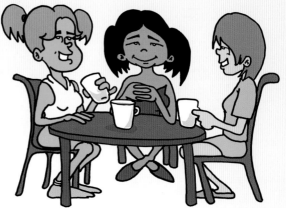

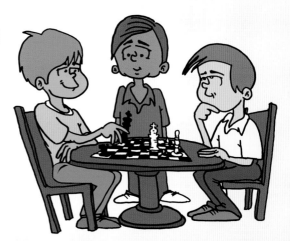

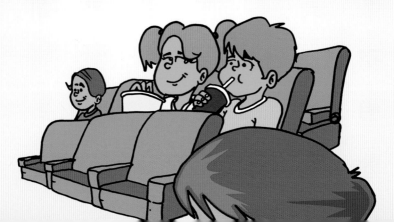

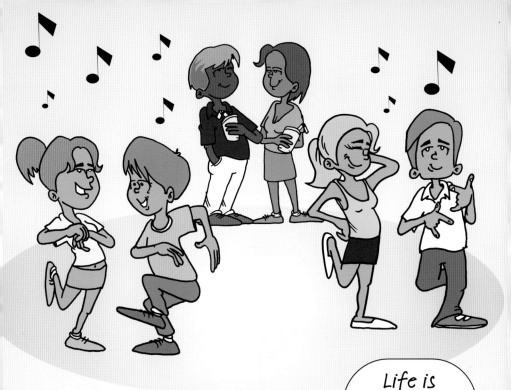

Some people take time to form friendships while others make new friends quickly.

Many young people find it easier to form friendships while participating in group activities such as chess club, team sports or part-time work.

It is normal to sometimes feel lonely or awkward when joining a new group. Some groups are easier to join because the members are welcoming and friendly.

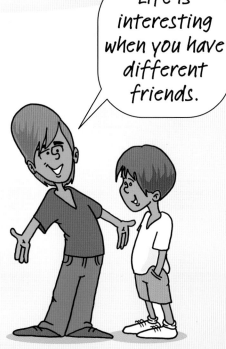

Life is interesting when you have different friends.

FRIENDSHIP CHECKLIST

Fun to be with ☑

Likes doing similar things ☑

Doesn't put me down ☑

Makes me feel safe ☑

Helps me be a confident person ☑

Treats me with respect ☑

Listens to me ☑

Doesn't push me around ☑

Understands my point of view ☑

Shares and takes turns in
what we do ☑

Talks about things so we make
decisions together ☑

Negotiates choices ☑

Together we make a good team ☑

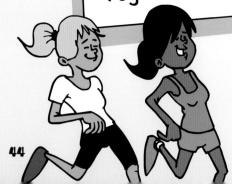

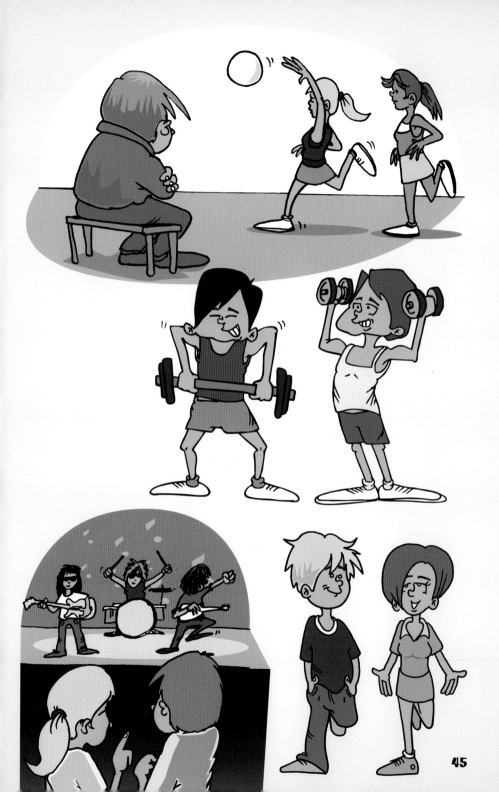

45

Friendship issues

It's normal for friends to disagree sometimes or say things that might hurt the other person's feelings.

However, if this happens often it may cause unhappiness and stress.

What can help

- Talk to the friend about your feelings.
- Listen carefully to your friend's response.
- Have the courage to tell a friend politely if they have done something or said something that annoyed you or hurt your feelings.

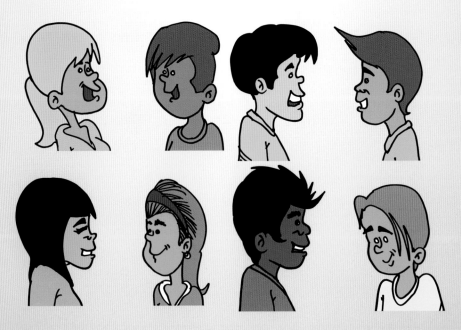

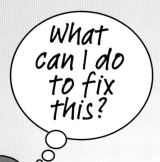

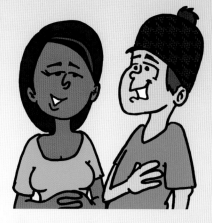

- If you have annoyed or hurt a friend's feelings, apologise, and work out how you can avoid doing the same thing in future.
- Check if you are both doing all the things on the 'Friendship Checklist'.
- Talk to a trusted adult, a parent, a teacher or school counsellor.

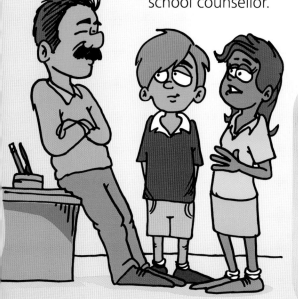

If these things have been tried and things haven't improved, it might be time to be less involved with that person and explore new friendships.

Is this a crush?
Am I falling in love?

At puberty there is an increase in romantic and sexual thoughts and feelings. Hormones are responsible for these changes.

Some people will have romantic or sexual feelings early in puberty while others will have these feelings later or maybe not at all. This means that in a group of friends, some may be really interested in having a romantic relationship, while others are not.

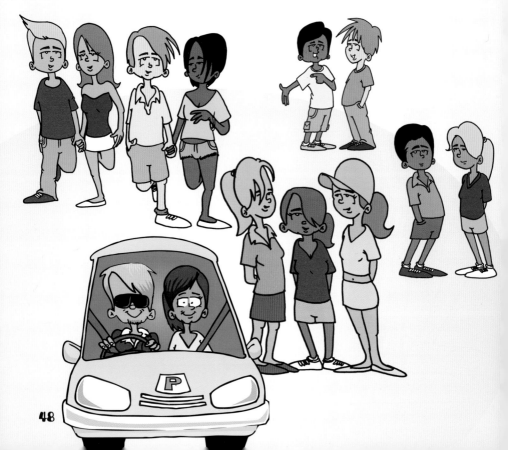

Young people might find that they are attracted to another person in a new way. They may spend a lot of time thinking about them, have butterflies in the tummy if they meet, and daydream about kissing and cuddling.

Young people might have a 'crush' on a football star, actor, member of a band or a teacher, but would never expect to have a romantic relationship with that person.

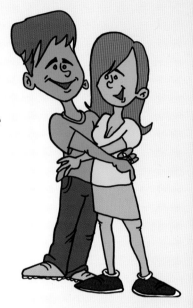

If a young person has a crush on someone of the same sex it does not necessarily mean they are gay. However some people will be naturally same-sex-attracted.

Some people may have inner feelings that they are the opposite sex to their body.

This can be a time of uncertainty and mixed emotions.

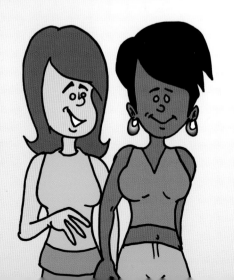

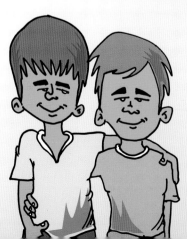

Gay or gender questioning

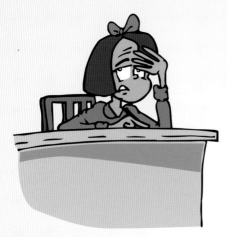

Some young people will be attracted to the opposite sex, some to the same sex or both sexes, and others will be undecided or feel no sexual attraction at all. Some people may feel that they are a different gender to their birth gender. Sometimes feelings change, go away or stay the same, and that's OK.

If a young person is wondering about their sexuality they may have different feelings: curiosity, excitement, confusion, embarrassment, loneliness or sadness. They might believe that they are different from everybody else. They may be confused about whether they should let others know or keep it a secret. There can be fears of rejection and loss of self-esteem.

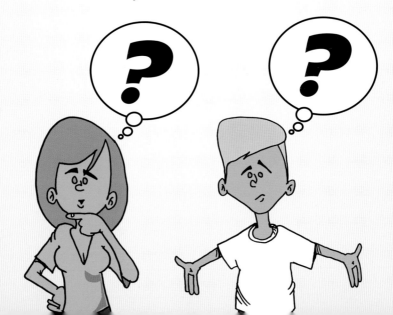

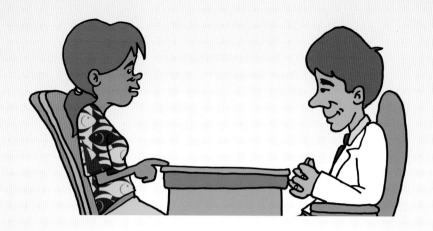

In the past, gay people rarely talked publicly about their sexuality. Now many gay people 'come out' in public and are willing to share their experiences. This can be positive and helpful for young people.

Young people 'come out' when they feel safe to do so, but some young people will never talk about their sexuality publicly. This is OK. Coming out needs to be thought about carefully: when, how and to whom. Support from friends, family, counsellors and professionals is extremely helpful.

There is support available for young people who are questioning their sexuality or gender. Counsellors, Kids Helpline or doctors will provide guidance and assistance.

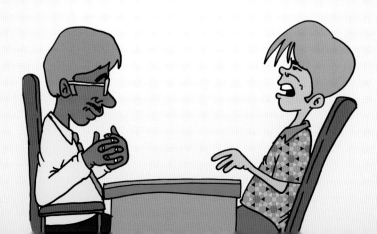

Same sex attracted and gender diverse

Sexual diversity is normal variation in human sexual development. GLBTIQ is a short way of describing sexual diversity. It stands for:

- **G**ay: A person who is romantically or sexually attracted to someone of the same sex.

- **L**esbian: A female who is romantically or sexually attracted to another female.

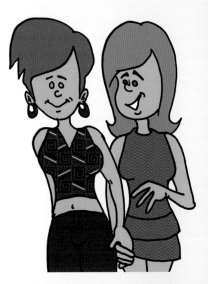

- **B**isexual: A person who is romantically or sexually attracted to both males and females.

- **T**ransgender: A person who has an inner feeling that they are the opposite sex to their body.

- **I**ntersex people are born with genetic, hormonal or physical (internal or external genitalia) features that are:
  - Not wholly female or male.
  - A combination of female and male.
  - Neither female nor male.

- **Q**ueer: gay, lesbian, bisexual and transgender people may choose to describe themselves as queer or gender queer.

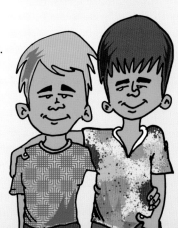

Some people may also be:

- Asexual: someone who does not experience sexual attraction. Unlike celibacy, when people choose not to have sexual relations, asexuality is an intrinsic part of the person.

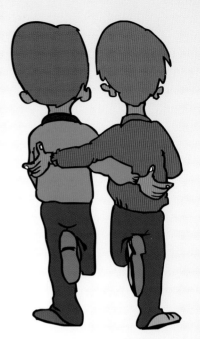

It is never appropriate to show negative feelings to someone because of their sexuality or gender. There are many differences in the way people develop, including their sexuality. Everyone deserves respect, no matter what their sexuality.

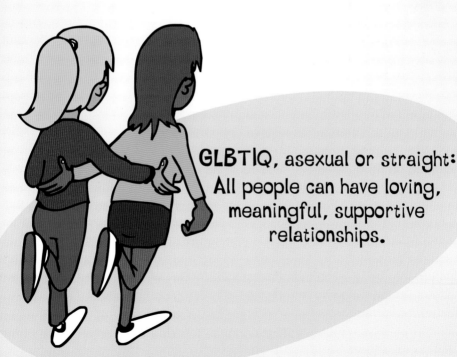

GLBTIQ, asexual or straight: All people can have loving, meaningful, supportive relationships.

Discrimination and harassment

Discrimination and harassment means being treated unfairly or picked on because of gender, religious beliefs, disability, race, colour, age, sexuality or marital status. In Australia, laws protect all people from discrimination and harassment.

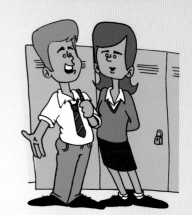

Some people, including GLBTIQ people, may experience harassment and discrimination.

This can be distressing, isolating, depressing and at times terrifying.

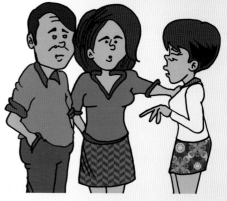

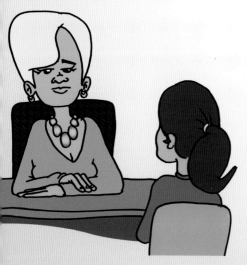

Ways to deal with harassment:

- Tell a trusted friend.
- Tell an adult, parents or a teacher.
- Report it to someone in authority for example a teacher, boss, or a manager.
- Call a counselling service.
- Report it to the police.

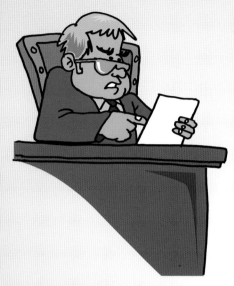

Discrimination and harassment is against the law, whether people are at school, TAFE or university, at work, unemployed, playing sport, or using social media.

There are many differences in the way people develop, including their sexuality. It is never appropriate to show negative feelings to someone because of their sexuality or gender.

EVERYONE DESERVES RESPECT!

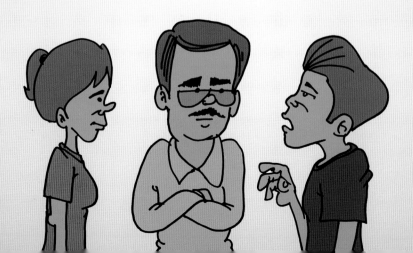

Relationships

Whatever their sexual orientation, people seek to form relationships with others.

Flirting

Flirting is lighthearted fun behavior that attracts attention and sparks someone's interest.

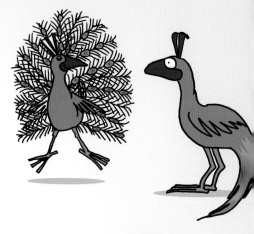

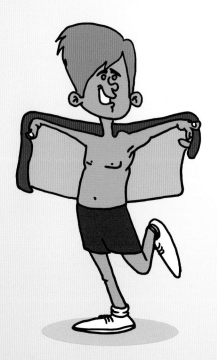

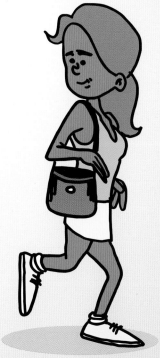

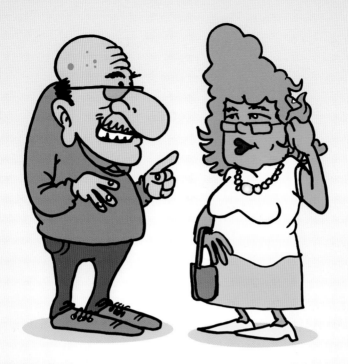

Flirting often takes place through texting, social media, on-line chat and messaging.

Face-to-face flirting behavior may include:
- talking, giggling or laughing more loudly,
- making jokes, gentle teasing,
- being happy and playful,
- flicking hair,
- making eye contact, fluttering eyelashes,
- standing or sitting closer than usual,
- walking to attract,
- dressing to impress.

Flirting is common between people of all ages who are attracted to each other.

Showing you're interested

If a young person is attracted to someone and wants to let them know, they can:

- Start by flirting a little.
- Smile and act in a friendly way.
- Talk about things they find interesting.
- Spend time together in a group.

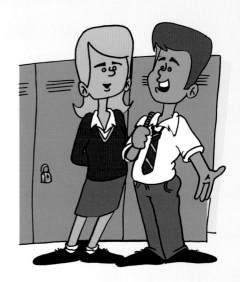

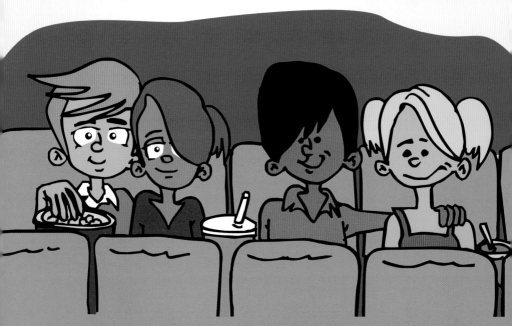

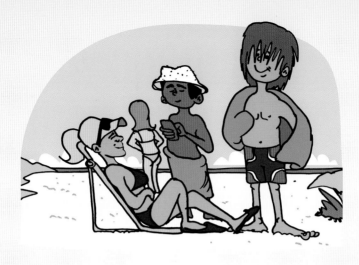

- Be casual and relaxed and not too pushy or obvious.
- Invite them to do something as a couple, e.g. have a coffee.
- Tell them you really like them.

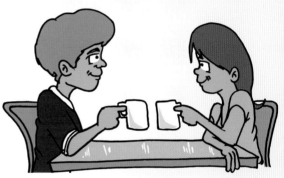

- Send a friendly text message or email.
- Check if they are going out with anyone else.

If the attraction is mutual, a romantic relationship may develop.

If this does not happen, be prepared to 'move on' and not be too disappointed. Maybe that friend was not ready for a romantic relationship.

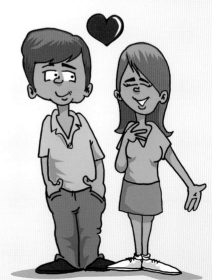

BEGINNING A ROMANTIC RELATIONSHIP

If your friend is romantically interested in you, you could:

- Arrange to spend more time together.
- Phone, chat online or send text messages.
- Hold hands.
- Sit close together for a private chat.
- Go to the movies together.
- Do homework together.

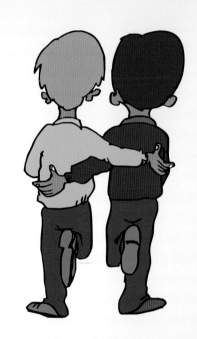

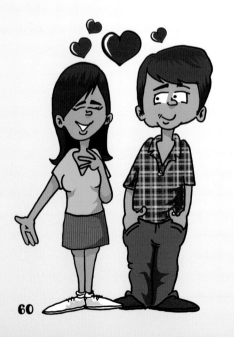

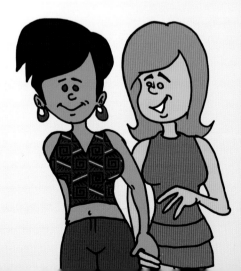

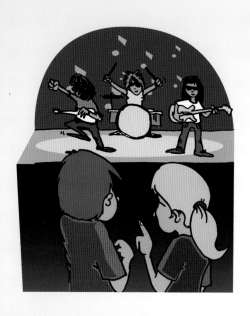

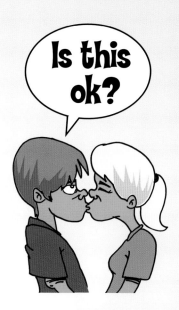

- Travel to school together or walk home together.
- Put your arm around his/her shoulder.
- Dance together.
- Cuddle in front of the TV.
- Kiss.

It is important to be thoughtful about physical approaches as some people do not want to hold hands, hug or be kissed. It may be too soon or they may not like it.

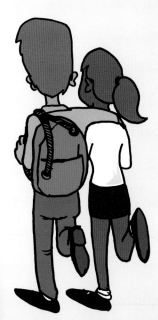

Think carefully about what you tell your friends about your relationship. Some people may later regret sharing private information.

SEEING SOMEONE, GOING OUT, DATING

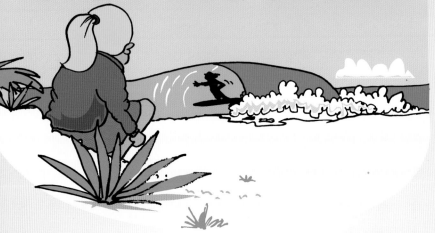

The first romantic relationship may be fun and exciting, but at the same time there may be feelings of uncertainty and a lack of confidence.

Established friends may feel left out and it can be tricky getting the balance right. Ideally there will be time for the new relationship whilst maintaining existing friendships.

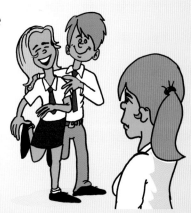

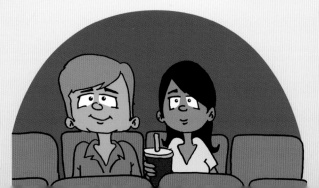

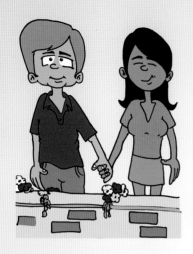
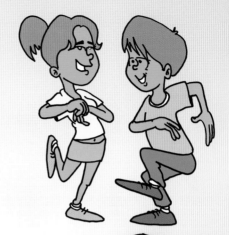

Relationships work well when couples :

- Care for and about each other.
- Listen to each other thoughtfully.
- Can talk about very personal matters.
- Trust each other.
- Respect each other's feeling and beliefs.
- Respect the privacy of their relationship.
- Enjoy being physically close, kissing, hugging and snuggling.

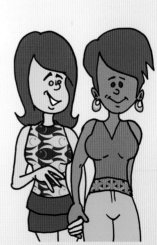

It's normal for first romantic relationships to last for a short time. This may be a number of days, weeks or months. Young people may have several relationships before they have a more permanent one.

Some people will have a number of romantic relationships in their teens and for others it will be later. Having a romantic relationship is only one aspect of a full happy life.

ROCKY TIMES!

If the relationship is not working

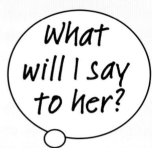

What will I say to her?

Many young people are unsure how they can end a relationship in a kind way that causes the least amount of hurt to the other person.

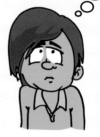

Breaking up in a respectful way takes a lot of courage.

It may help to practice a few times and think carefully about:

☆ What to say.
☆ When is the best time.
☆ Where to have the conversation.

Most people would rather be told about a relationship break-up in a direct, respectful manner, face-to-face, or perhaps over the phone. To get the message by text, email or from other people can be embarrassing or hurtful.

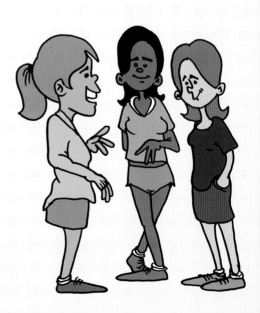

Some examples of what to say

'I'm not ready for a relationship.'

'You are a really nice person but I don't want to "go" with you any more.'

'I was really hurt when you did that, and I don't want to go with you any longer.'

'I know this will hurt you but I need to tell you that I have met someone else.'

'This is not about you as a person, but I no longer have romantic feelings for you.'

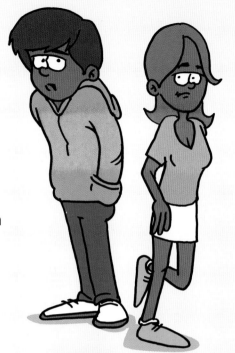

Be prepared for the other person to be upset, cry or be angry.

Think about how *you* would prefer to hear about a break-up. This may help to decide the best way to break-up.

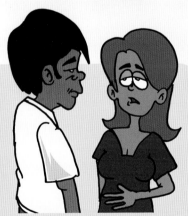

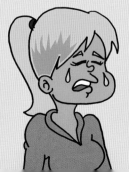

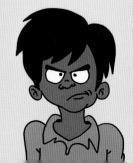

Dealing with a relationship break-up

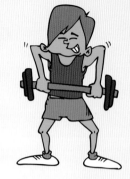

Most people have had broken relationships during their life. Here are some hints to help deal with this difficult time.

⚡ Know that it is OK to be upset.

⚡ Try to avoid your 'ex' if you can.

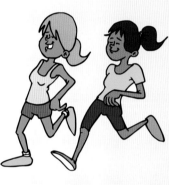

⚡ Avoid the temptation to criticize your 'ex' to friends or family.

⚡ Don't post private information about your breakup on social media!

⚡ Look after yourself. Make sure you eat regular meals and get enough sleep.

⚡ Keep busy, plan fun activities with friends or family.

⚡ Do things you enjoy such as listening to music that makes you feel happier, reading, watching movies, playing sport.

⚡ Don't put yourself down. The end of a relationship doesn't mean there is anything wrong with you.

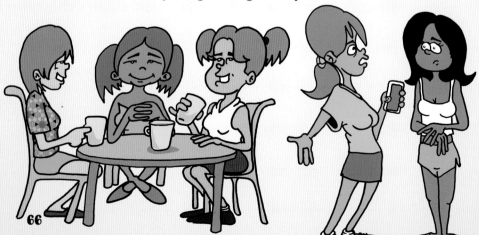

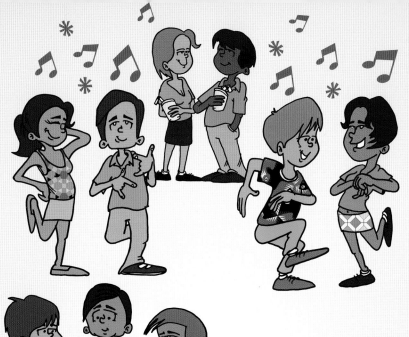

You won't feel like this forever. These feelings of sadness will slowly fade.

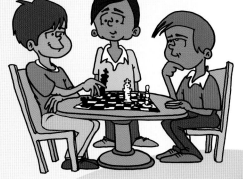

If feelings of sadness persist you need to discuss this with a doctor.

Learn from this experience and think about what you want in a future relationship.

Give yourself time, don't rush into a new relationship, enjoy being single.

Ongoing relationships – Making out, fooling around

If a relationship grows and develops, couples may be ready to become sexually closer.

There are many things they can do when they are 'making out' or 'fooling around'.

Some of these are:

Holding hands, touching or stroking hair, giggling, kissing, whispering words of love, cuddling, touching breasts, kissing the neck, caressing, lying on top of each other with clothes on, stroking each other's bodies, tongue kissing, touching each other's genitals, oral sex.

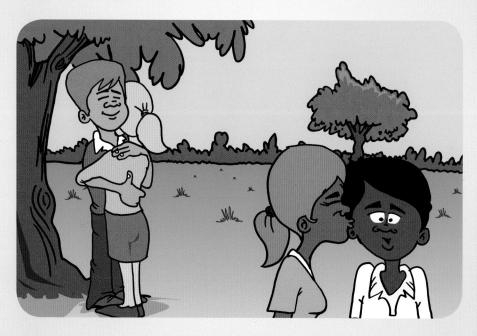

Some couples may decide to have sexual intercourse. Some people will choose to do this early in a relationship, others will wait until they know each other very well and both feel comfortable and ready. Some other couples will wait until after they are married before they have sex.

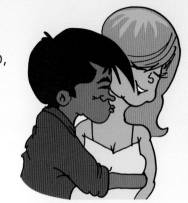

Each person is an individual, and their attitude to sex before marriage is influenced by many factors including their family values, culture and religion. This can be a worthwhile discussion to have with a partner.

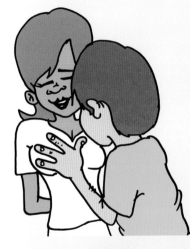

Many young people will be happy to 'make out' for several months or years.

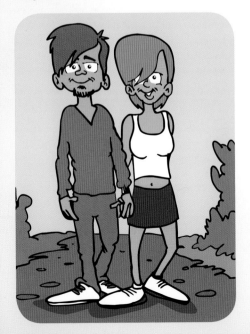

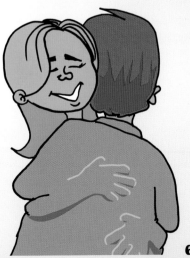

Consent

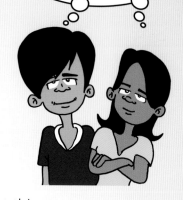

It's my decision who touches me and how and where it happens.

Consent means to agree to, give permission, or allow something.

People in a relationship should feel free to say what they like, or want to happen, and what they don't like or don't want to happen. This is giving consent. It's OK to say 'Stop, I don't like it!' This is their right, and a caring partner will respect this.

Ongoing consent for any sexual behavior is essential. Check with your partner often. People may agree to try something but then want to stop. They may feel OK about doing some things today but not tomorrow and that is OK.

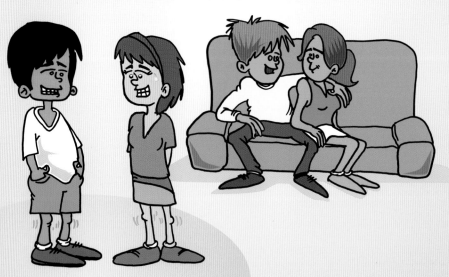

Some helpful questions are:
'Is this OK?'
'Do you like me doing this?'
'Do you want me to stop?'

Be sensitive to non-verbal cues and body language:

- Is your partner's body tense or relaxed?
- Are they holding you or pushing you away?
- Are they looking happy, upset? Turned on or disinterested?

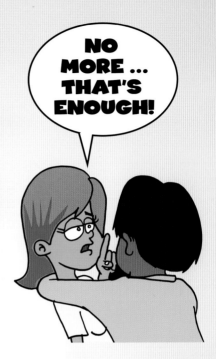

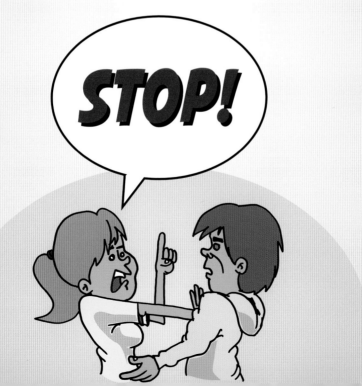

SeXUAL FeeLINGS

The sex drive is a powerful natural instinct that develops after puberty and ensures the continuation of the human race. It is a strong urge to be closer to someone and to have sex.

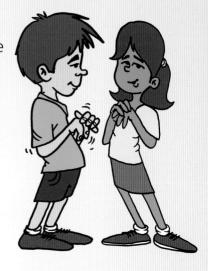

Sexual arousal brings about:
- Warm, tingly, exciting feelings in the body.
- Increase in heart and breathing rates.
- Skin more sensitive to touch.
- Nipples harden.
- The penis becomes erect.
- The vagina lubricates.
- Urge to have sexual intercourse is felt.

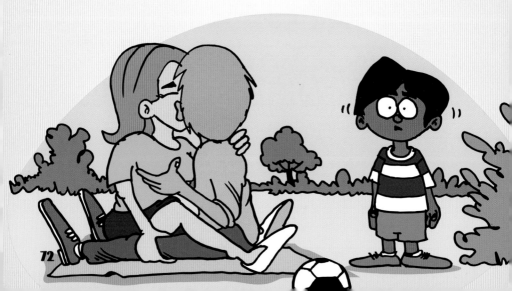

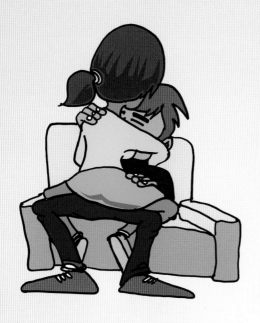

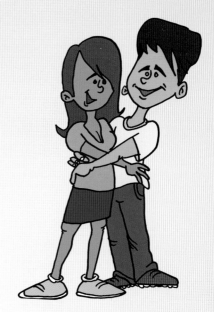

The sex drive can surprise people by developing quickly and powerfully in some situations, such as standing close together, hugging or kissing.

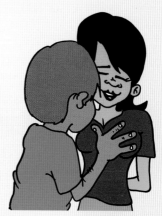

Sexual arousal may last for a few minutes or even several hours. Just because someone is sexually aroused doesn't mean they must have sex. Sexual arousal can fade with time, or be relieved by masturbation.

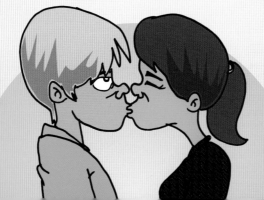

Having sex - your decision

Although a person may be sexually aroused, this does not necessarily mean that it is the right time to have sex or that they are emotionally ready.

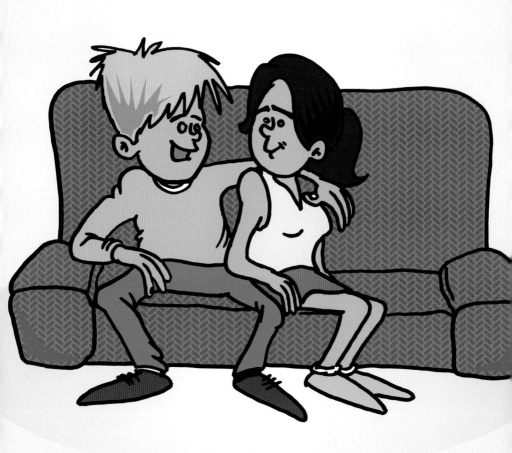

There are important things to consider **before** deciding if a relationship becomes sexual. *It is **much** easier to think about this before an intimate situation develops.*

Think carefully about the relationship, and the positives and negatives of having sex, before deciding if the time is right.

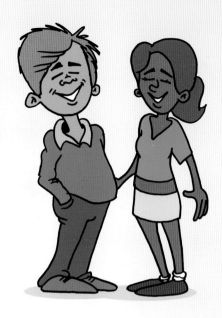

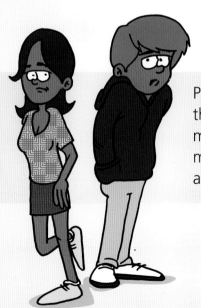

People who have sex without thinking about it beforehand may have regrets later. They may feel disappointed, guilty, ashamed or upset.

Choosing not to have sex

Young people might decide not to have sex for any of the following reasons:

- They might not be old enough to have sex legally.
- Their personal values or beliefs may be that it is wrong to have sex before marriage.
- They might be under the influence of drugs or alcohol. This is not a good time to make such an important decision.
- One person may not have clearly given consent, and may feel pressured.
- They will lose their 'virginity' and might wish they had waited.
- Risk of pregnancy and STIs.
- Worry that they will not know what to do, which could be embarrassing.

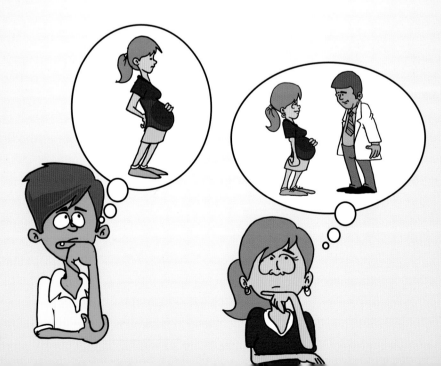

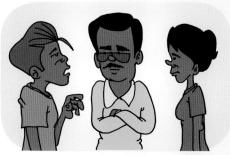

- It might not be 'special' or enjoyable.
- Fear of being hurt emotionally or physically.
- Worry about how their sexual partner will behave afterwards.
- Parents might find out and be upset.

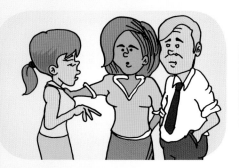

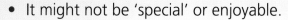

- May feel 'used' if the relationships doesn't last.
- Location may not be comfortable, private or safe.
- Can't trust their partner to keep the relationship private.

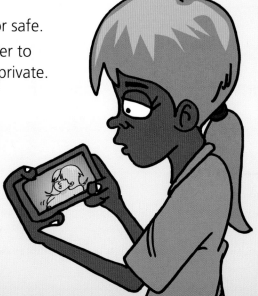

Saying 'No' to sex – getting the message across

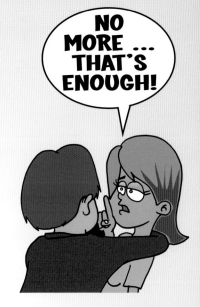

- Tell the other person clearly and firmly, 'I do not want to have sex'.
- State that, 'Sex without consent is against the law'.
- Move away, put some distance between you.
- If clothes have been removed, get dressed.
- State clearly. 'I want to go home' or 'I want to go back to my friends'.
- Walk to another room or a place where there are other people around.
- Phone a friend, parents or another adult, or call a taxi.

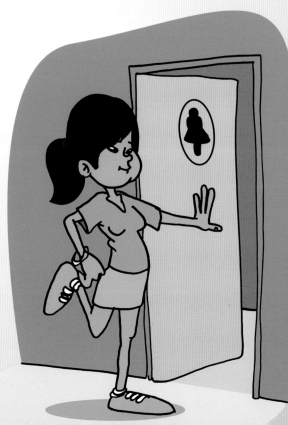

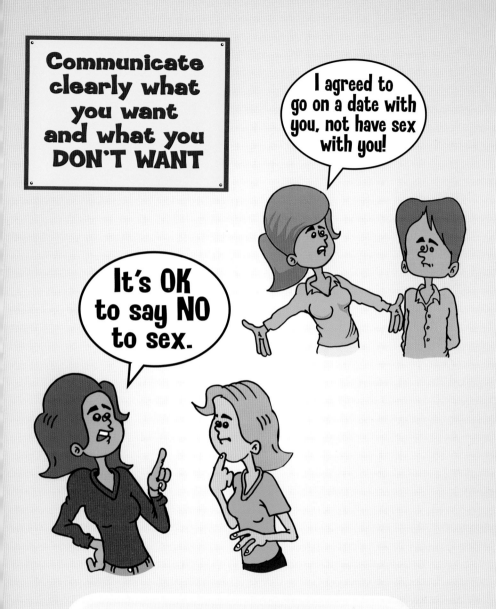

Choosing to have sex

Couples might decide to have sex because:

- ❤ They care about or love each other.
- ❤ They enjoy being physically close, kissing and hugging, and are sexually aroused by each other.
- ❤ It feels 'right' for both people and they both feel ready.
- ❤ They can communicate freely and openly.
- ❤ Both people have clearly consented and understand the law.

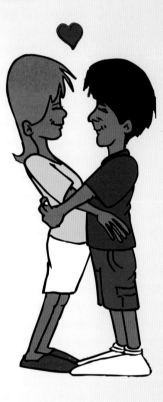

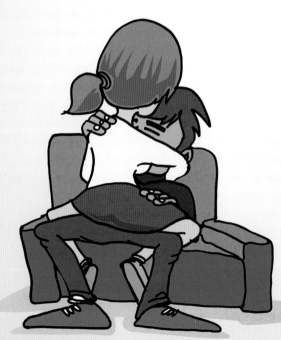

- They have made a thoughtful decision, not effected by drugs and alcohol.
- Having sex may develop and strengthen the relationship.
- They respect each other's feelings and beliefs.
- They respect the privacy of the relationship.
- Both will share responsibility for contraception and prevention of STIs.

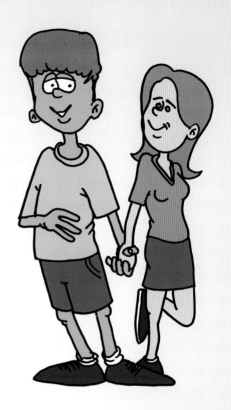

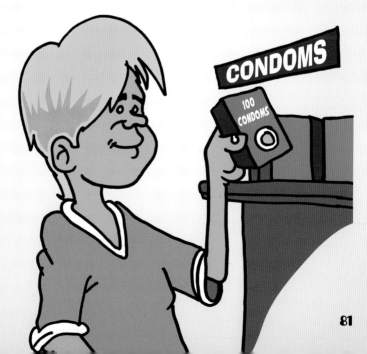

CONDOMS

100 CONDOMS

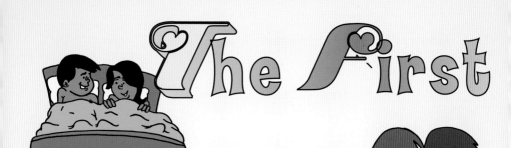

The First

First experiences of sex vary greatly due to many factors, including:

 ## Location

Somewhere comfortable, private and safe to be together.

 ## Thoughts and feelings

Embarrassment, worry and uncertainty can mean that people do not relax. This may prevent arousal and cause muscles to tighten. The vagina may not lubricate, the penis might not be fully erect: these things make intercourse uncomfortable and difficult.

 ## Body image

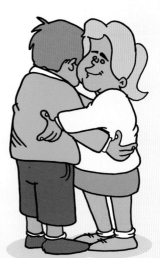

Both males and females may worry about the look and size of their bodies and their genitals.

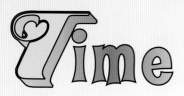

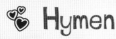 Hymen

Girls are born with a thin layer of skin (hymen) just inside the vaginal opening. The hymen stretches as they grow and the small holes in it enlarge during normal activities such as running and jumping. During first sexual intercourse any remaining hymen may tear, stinging a little and causing a small amount of bleeding.

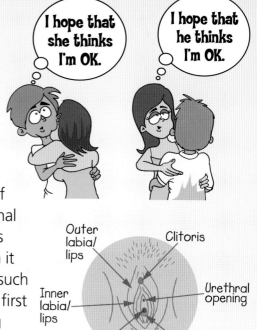

Outer labial/lips

Clitoris

Inner labial/lips

Urethral opening

Vaginal opening

Hymen

Lubrication

Water-based lubricant from the supermarket or chemist can be applied to the vagina or penis to make sex more comfortable.

Afterwards

Afterwards, there may be some discomfort in the genitals from rubbing and stretching of the soft skin. It is helpful to pass urine (have a wee) soon after sex as this may prevent urinary tract infections.

If it's the right time, the right partner, the right place, the right decision there is more chance sex will be enjoyable the first time.

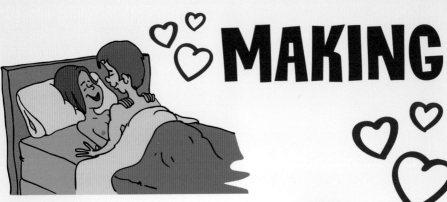

MAKING

Foreplay

Foreplay may include kissing, whispering words of love, caressing each other's bodies or mutual masturbation. It increases sexual arousal and prepares the body for having sexual intercourse, making the experience more pleasurable. The penis becomes erect and the vagina becomes lubricated.

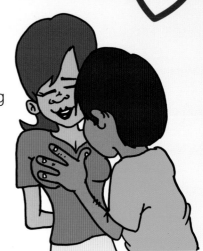

Male-female sexual intercourse

The penis slides into the vagina. Their bodies move together and the penis rubs against the inside of the vagina. This should feel pleasurable for both the male and female. They may breathe loudly or make noises.

With practice, couples learn what gives them and their partner the greatest pleasure.

LOVE

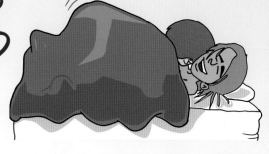

These sexual feelings increase until the male orgasms and ejaculates. The penis then returns to normal size. Some young males may ejaculate quickly but can get an erection again soon after sex.

Women's sexual response varies greatly. If the clitoris is stimulated sufficiently during sexual intercourse an orgasm may occur. Some women will orgasm before or after sex when their clitoris is stimulated by their partner or themselves.

What if I'm 'GLBTIQ'?

As with 'straight' couples, GLBTIQ couples cuddle, kiss and discuss what will give each other sexual pleasure. All people, regardless of their sexuality, sexual preference, or gender identity, can have loving and satisfying sexual relationships.

After sex, people usually feel warm, happy, relaxed and loving, and enjoy being emotionally and physically close to their partner.

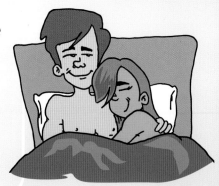

Note: The enjoyment of sex generally increases with experience, good communication, enjoyable foreplay and understanding how your partner responds sexually.

PREVENTING PREGNANCY – CONTRACEPTION

Young people's bodies are very efficient at ensuring that sperm unite with an egg to make a baby.

The following factors combine to achieve the best possible chance of pregnancy occurring:

- Powerful sexual feelings
- Millions of sperm in each ejaculation
- In females, fertile mucus helps draw the sperm to the ripening egg.

There are, however, a number of ways to prevent fertilization. This is called 'contraception'. A good understanding of this helps to avoid pregnancy.

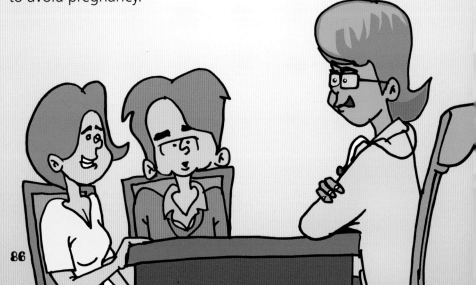

Some common methods of contraception are:

The oral contraceptive pill

One pill is taken every day at approximately the same time.

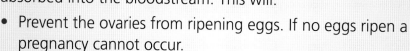

The pill contains hormones that are absorbed into the bloodstream. This will:

- Prevent the ovaries from ripening eggs. If no eggs ripen a pregnancy cannot occur.
- Change the lining of the uterus and prevent a fertilized egg from embedding.
- Thicken the mucus at the cervix, stopping sperm from getting through.

The pill is a safe and reliable form of contraception if it is taken as instructed.

The pill may not work if:

- it is not taken every day,
- vomiting or diarrhoea has occurred,
- antibiotics are being taken.

A doctor, nurse or pharmacist can advise about this and may recommend emergency contraception.

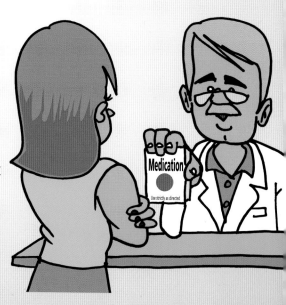

Hormone implant

A small, thin, soft rod of plastic is inserted by a trained doctor just under the skin on the inside of the female's upper arm. The rod contains the hormone progesterone that is slowly released over a 3 year period. The implant:

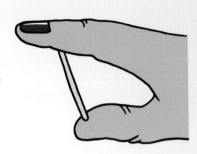

- Prevents the ovaries ripening eggs.
- Makes the lining of the uterus unsuitable for pregnancy.
- Thickens the mucus at the cervix to prevent sperm entering.

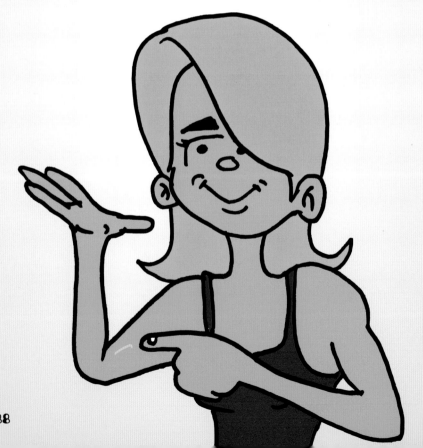

The implant is a very effective form of contraception that lasts for 3 years and does not rely on the user remembering to take a daily pill.

Some women who have the implant inserted do not have a period, which is OK. Some will have irregular spotting or bleeding which may be annoying. Some will discuss this with their doctor and have it removed.

In Australia a doctor can legally prescribe the pill or implant to girls over the age of 16, or under 16 if the doctor decides the girl understands how this contraception works and knows about possible side effects.

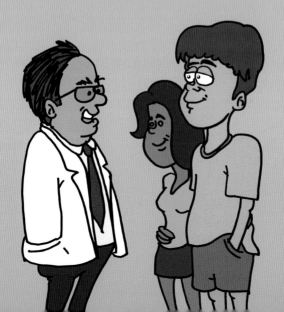

Condoms

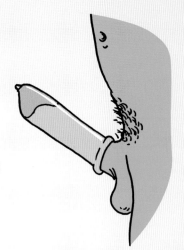

A condom is made of very thin rubber that rolls down over the penis. During ejaculation, semen is caught in the end of the condom. Condoms are effective if used correctly but sometimes they can slip off or break.

Condom hints

- Store condoms in a cool place to prevent deterioration of the rubber.
- Check the use-by date on the packet.
- Take great care not to tear the condom when opening the packet. Teeth and fingernails can damage condoms.
- Squeeze air out of the tip of the condom so that there is room for the semen.
- Make sure the roll is on the outside so the condom will roll down the penis easily.

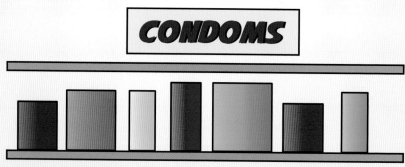

A wide range of colours, sizes, textures and flavours
6-pack, 12-pack, 24-pack, ribbed, ticklers

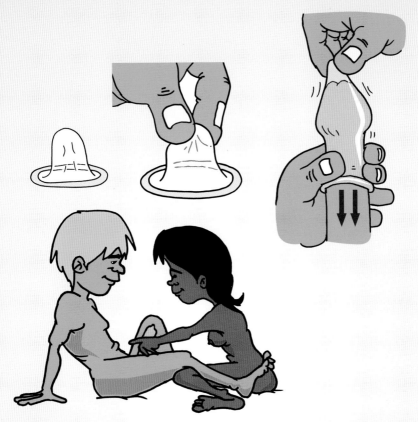

- Put the condom on the penis before any genital contact.
- After ejaculation, hold the condom firmly at the base of the penis while it is withdrawn from the vagina. Do this before the penis becomes smaller and softens, to avoid spilling semen.
- Water based lubricant can be used for extra comfort and helps to prevent condom breakage. Do not use saliva, Vaseline, baby oil, cooking oil or body lotion as these can damage condoms.
- Don't wear two condoms at once. Friction between the condoms can cause them to break.

Dispose of used condoms in the rubbish bin. Do not flush them down the toilet or leave them lying around.

The female condom

The female condom is made of polyurethane and is inserted into the vagina before sex. It provides a barrier between the penis and the vagina and prevents sperm from entering the uterus, preventing pregnancy and the spread of STIs.

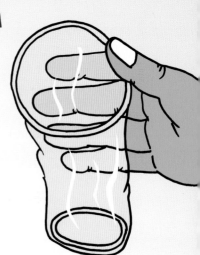

Emergency contraception – the Morning After Pill

This hormone tablet can help prevent pregnancy after unprotected sex, which may occur during a sexual assault (e.g. no condom, broken condom or missed pills). It prevents ovulation and makes the lining of the uterus unsuitable for pregnancy. It works best if it is taken as soon as possible after unprotected sex and becomes less effective as time passes. It may still work up to 1 week later. In Australia it can be bought from the pharmacy with no age restriction.

Contraception – Whose responsibility?

Some people believe it's up to the female, some people believe it's up to the male to ensure that contraception is used. The fact is, it takes two to have sex, so it must be a shared responsibility.

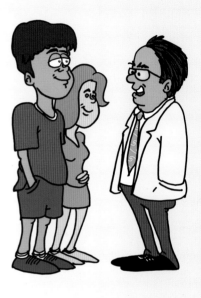

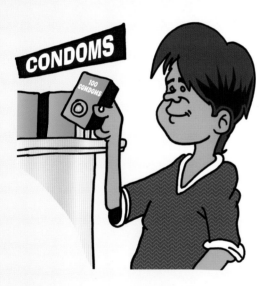

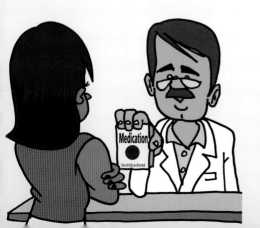

Talk to a doctor about the most effective method of contraception.

SOME UNRELIABLE FORMS

The Withdrawal Method

This form of contraception relies on the male being able to pull his penis out of the vagina (withdraw) before he ejaculates. This control can be tricky, especially for young males. Another risk factor is that when a male is sexually aroused, 'pre-cum' on the tip of the penis may contain sperm.

The withdrawal method is definitely not a reliable way to prevent pregnancy.

OF CONTRACEPTION

Time of the Month (Rhythm Method or Calendar Method)

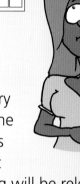

Oh! No... my period is late!

Some couples try to prevent pregnancy by not having sex around the time of ovulation. However it is very difficult to predict when ovulation will occur. A woman's cycle can vary greatly due to many things including hormone changes, stress or illness. As ovulation occurs 12–16 days *before* the *next* period, it is not possible to accurately calculate when the egg will be released. After ovulation, the egg lives for two days. Another important factor is that sperm can live for 5 days inside the vagina or uterus. This makes it extremely difficult to predict when conception is possible. Consequently, the calendar method is not reliable.

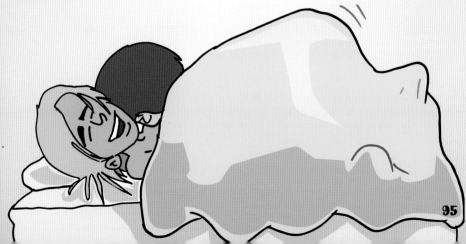

Contraception myths

There are many myths and misunderstandings about contraception.

Here are some examples.

Pregnancy will not happen if:

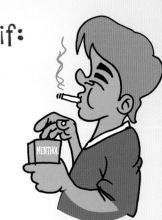

- It's the first time you have had sex. *This is not true.*
- The penis is withdrawn from the vagina before ejaculation. *This is not true.*
- Menthol cigarettes are smoked. *This is not true.*
- The female does/does not orgasm during sex. *This is not true.*
- Sex takes place while standing up. *This is not true.*
- The female jumps up and down after sex. *This is not true.*
- The vagina is washed out after sex. *This is not true.*

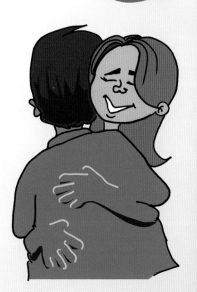

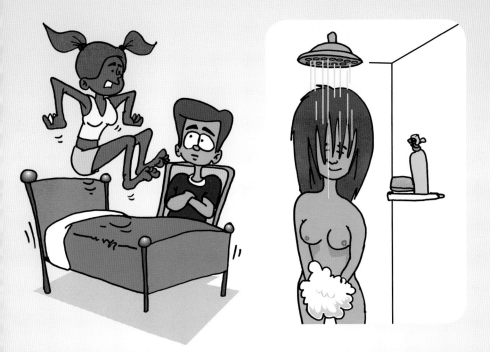

- Sex takes place during the period. *This is not true.*
- Contraception is used. *This is not true.*
  - *Contraception sometimes fails.*
- The male ejaculates outside the vagina. *This is not true.*
  - *Any sperm ejaculated near the vaginal entrance can track up the vagina and fertilise an egg.*

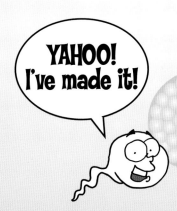

Unplanned pregnancy

There are times when no contraception is used or contraception fails and an unplanned pregnancy is the result.

This can come as a *huge* shock to both the female and the male.

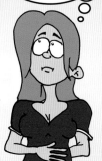

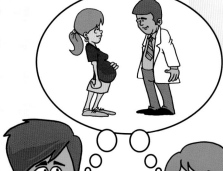

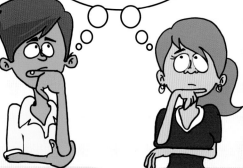

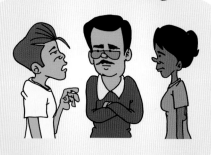

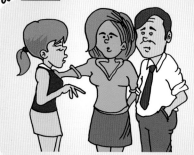

Early signs of pregnancy

In the first months of pregnancy many females notice changes in their feelings and their body. They may notice:

- A missed period or unusually light period.
- Tiredness.
- Breasts swollen, tender or sore.
- Need to wee more often.
- Nausea, or 'morning sickness'.
- Sensitivity to some tastes and smells.

However, some pregnant women do not notice any physical or emotional signs.

Pregnancy tests

If a young woman thinks that there is any chance that she might be pregnant, it is important to buy a 'do it yourself' pregnancy test or go to the doctor for a test as soon as possible. Anyone can buy a pregnancy test from the chemist or supermarket. Early morning urine gives more accurate test results.

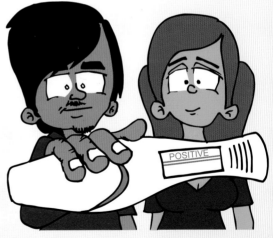

If the test result is negative but a period has been missed, it is important to see the doctor, as there could still be a chance of pregnancy.

An appointment with the doctor

As soon as a period is late it is time to visit the doctor or family planning clinic if there is a chance of pregnancy.

The doctor will:

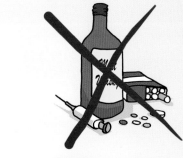

- Confirm the pregnancy (tell the female if she is pregnant or not).
- Provide advice and support.
- Arrange blood and urine tests.
- Organize an ultrasound.
- Discuss pregnancy choices.
- Provide information about ways to protect the health of the developing baby. It is important to eat certain foods and avoid others. Cigarettes, alcohol and drugs can affect the health of the developing baby.

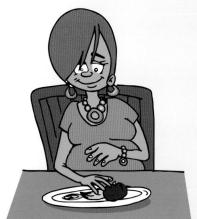

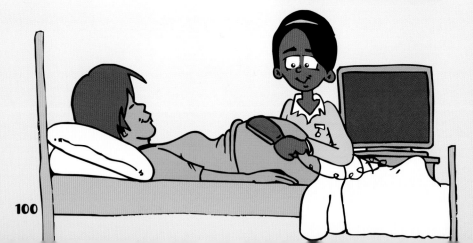

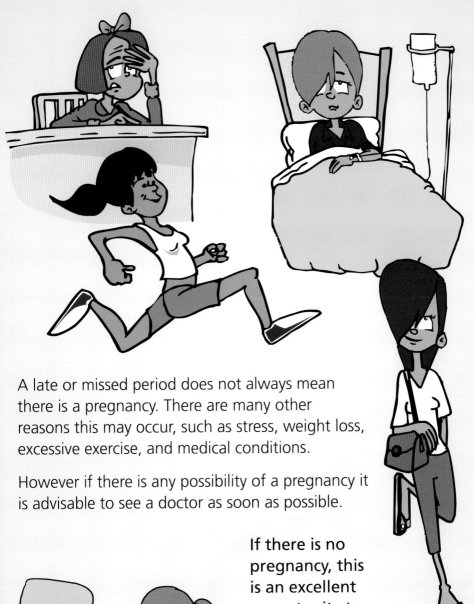

A late or missed period does not always mean there is a pregnancy. There are many other reasons this may occur, such as stress, weight loss, excessive exercise, and medical conditions.

However if there is any possibility of a pregnancy it is advisable to see a doctor as soon as possible.

If there is no pregnancy, this is an excellent opportunity to discuss ongoing contraception.

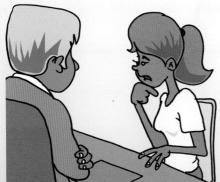

PREGNANCY CHOICES

If an unplanned pregnancy is confirmed, this can be overwhelming and distressing for a time. A young woman has the following choices:

- Continue the pregnancy.
- Continue the pregnancy and offer the baby for adoption.
- Terminate the pregnancy (abortion).

Making a decision can be very difficult. Counselling may be helpful. There needs to be a lot of careful thinking before a decision is made.

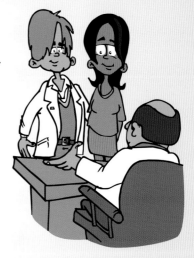

The father

Unplanned pregnancy is a big shock for the male as well as the female. He may have feelings of stress, guilt and concern. If they choose, the couple can visit the doctor together.

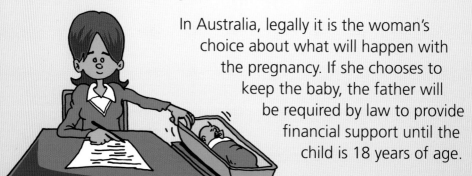

In Australia, legally it is the woman's choice about what will happen with the pregnancy. If she chooses to keep the baby, the father will be required by law to provide financial support until the child is 18 years of age.

Continuing the pregnancy

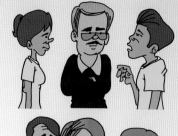

This will mean letting parents know. Yes, they will probably be upset initially, but they will most likely appreciate being told so they can help.

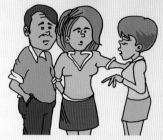

When deciding whether to continue with the pregnancy, consider the following:

- Does she feel ready and want to have a baby?
- Where will she live?
- How will she manage financially?

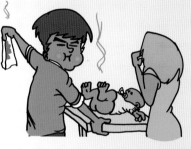

- Does she feel supported by the father or her family?
- Does she feel mature enough to provide for all the baby's needs?
- Does she want to continue her education and how could she do that?

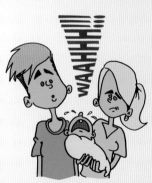

- Is she prepared to put her social life on hold for a while?

If these things have been considered and a decision has been made to go ahead with the pregnancy, there are many agencies to support young women before and after the birth. Agencies may provide pregnancy support, continuing education, training in parenting skills and also social activities.

Adoption

Choosing to have a baby adopted is a very difficult decision but in some circumstances it is the right choice for some women. A counsellor provides information and support throughout the adoption process.

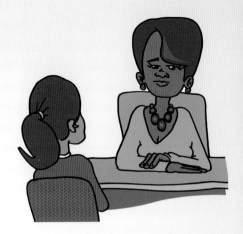

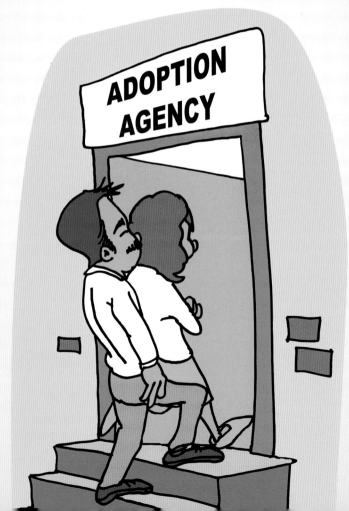

ADOPTION AGENCY

Termination of the pregnancy

Termination of a pregnancy is also described as an abortion.

It is usually a very hard decision to make but may be the right choice for some women.

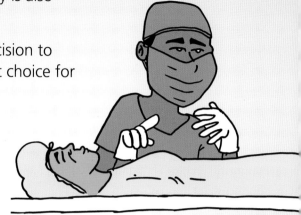

If the decision is made early in the pregnancy, medication can be used to bring about a 'medical abortion'. This is done under the care of a doctor.

More commonly, women choose a surgical abortion, which involves a small operation to remove the embryo from the uterus. This is best done before the 12th week of pregnancy.

Counselling is an essential part of decision-making about pregnancy choices.

This can be a time of shock, regret, guilt, helplessness, lack of control and worries about disappointing family and friends. Advice from well-meaning relatives and support people can be confusing.

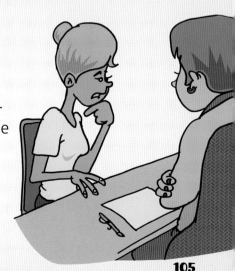

It is ultimately the young woman's choice, and is not appropriate for other people to pressure her or influence her decision.

Sexually transmitted infections (STIs)

Unprotected sex can result in unplanned pregnancy and STIs.

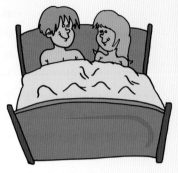

STIs are often not discussed, but it is very important to know about them. STIs are infections spread through sexual activity such as oral sex, sexual intercourse, anal sex or sharing sex toys.

There are many different types of STIs.

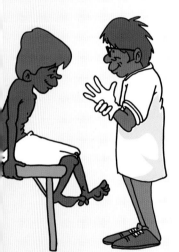

Bacterial STIs

e.g. chlamydia, syphilis, gonorrhoea

These bacterial STIs can easily be treated with antibiotics.

Chlamydia is common around the world and is the most common STI in Australia. Usually people do not know they have chlamydia, so it is often spread without people knowing. It can cause permanent damage to the fallopian tubes and infertility.

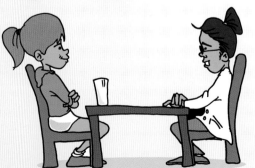

Viral STIs

e.g. genital warts, hepatitis, herpes, HIV/AIDS

This group of STIs generally cannot be cured but the symptoms can be treated. The virus stays in the body.

Note: Australia has a National Immunisation Program for 12–13 year-old boys and girls. This prevents genital warts that can cause cancer of the cervix, penis and anus.

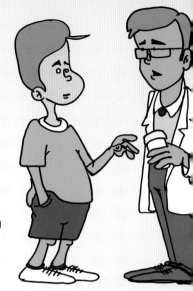

Other STIs

e.g. genital lice (crabs), thrush and scabies

These are more obvious because they are uncomfortable and unpleasant. These STIs can be easily treated with products purchased from a pharmacy.

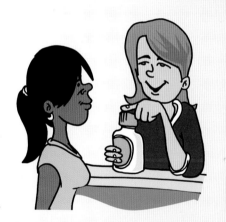

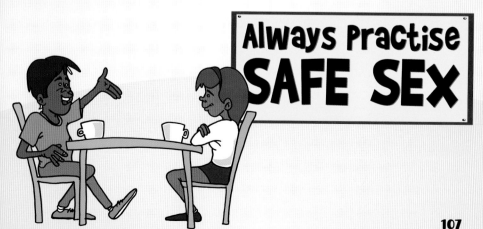

Always Practise SAFE SEX

Protection agains STIs

You can't always tell by looking at someone's body whether they have an STI. Many people with an STI have no symptoms.

To protect yourself from STIs:

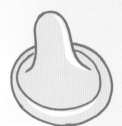

- Use a new condom every time sexual intercourse takes place
- Lubricant helps prevent condom breakage.
- For oral sex to males, use a condom
- For oral sex to females, place a dental dam over the vulva.
- Do not have sex with anyone if they tell you they have an STI or if you can see sores, ulcers or lumps in the genital or anal area.

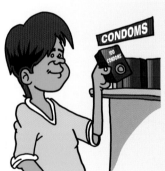

- Be aware STIs can be transmitted by sex toys.
- Explore other ways to be sexually intimate, such as kissing, cuddling, stroking, masturbation. These involve little risk of STIs and unplanned pregnancy.

Being in a loving, trusting relationship with someone who:

- you know does not have an STI, and
- does not have sex with anyone else,

is great protection against STIs.

When to have an STI check

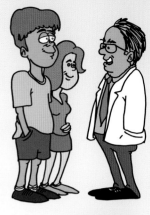

- If young people are sexually active, it is good to have an STI check by a doctor or at a Sexual Health Clinic.
- Before starting a new sexual relationship it is important for both partners to have a sexual health check.
- Any time a person is worried.
- If their partner has had sex with someone else.
- If there is a history of sexual abuse

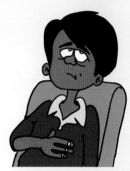

- If their partner or ex-partner says they have an STI.
- If the following symptoms develop:
  - vaginal discharge,
  - discharge from the penis,
  - sores, redness, rash or irritation in the genitals,
  - pain during sex,
  - pain or stinging during urination.

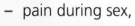

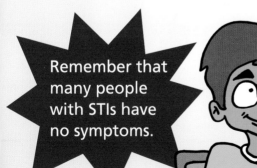

Remember that many people with STIs have no symptoms.

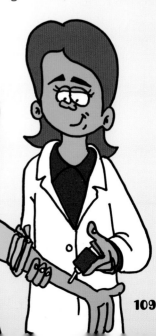

Sex and the Law

In most countries, laws have been written to protect children and young people from sexual assault or abuse.

Age of Consent

When an adult or young person engages in sexual behavior with someone below the 'age of consent', the adult is breaking the law. *The young person is not at fault and is not breaking the law*.

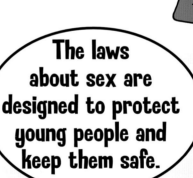

I have the right to FEEL SAFE around adults.

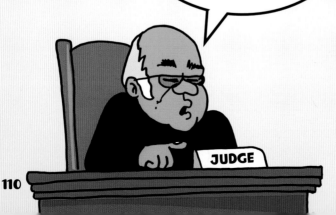

The laws about sex are designed to protect young people and keep them safe.

JUDGE

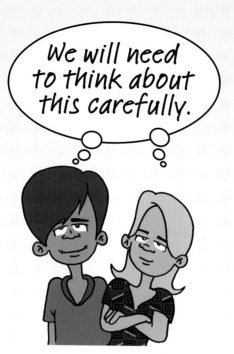

Laws about the age of consent are complicated! They vary in different states and countries.

In Australia, each state or Territory has its own laws about the age of consent. For example, the age of consent in the state of Victoria is 16 years of age. Check with your local Legal Aid Office or Community Legal Centre for information about laws in your area.

Note: At any age a person who is drunk, drug affected or unconscious cannot legally consent.

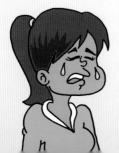

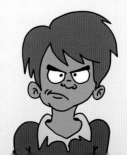

Sexual assault

Sexual assault is *ANY* unwanted sexual act or behaviour that is:

- persuasive, pressured, threatening, forced or violent,
- to which a person has not given consent or was not able to give consent (e.g. was unconscious, drunk, asleep, intellectually disabled).

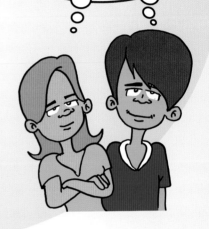

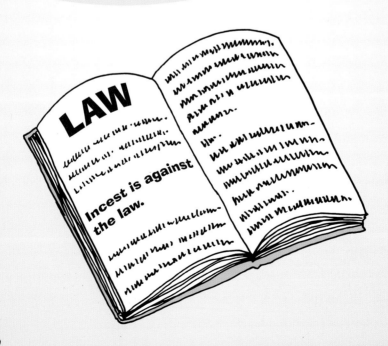

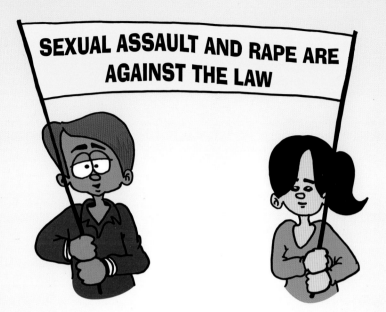

SEXUAL ASSAULT AND RAPE ARE AGAINST THE LAW

Examples of sexual assault include:

- Sexual harassment – making inappropriate sexual comments.
- Unwanted sexual touching.
- Showing pornographic pictures, DVDs or internet images.
- Exposing (showing) private parts.
- An older person asking a young person or child to touch them sexually.
- Being pressured to masturbate or forced to watch someone masturbate.
- Having sex.
- Putting a penis, other parts of the body or an object into someone's mouth, vagina or anus.
- Being forced to give or receive oral sex.

Sexual assault can be frightening, unexpected, traumatic, and sometimes violent or life threatening.

Sexual abuse

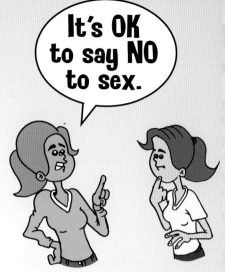

Sexual abuse is sexual assault which occurs when:

- Someone in a position of power or authority (e.g. a teacher), takes advantage of a person who trusts and respects them (e.g. a student), to involve them in sexual activity.

Sexual abuse can occur between:

- an adult and a child/young person,
- a young person and a child,
- a doctor and a patient,
- a priest and a young church-goer,
- a coach and a sports person.

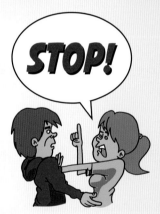

Incest

Incest is sex between a child and a family member (e.g. a parent, a step-parent, the partner of a parent, an older sibling, a grandparent, aunt, uncle or cousin). Incest is against the law. The child is not breaking the law, even if they consent. The adult or older person is breaking the law.

Sexual assault, sexual abuse and incest are crimes

Rape and date rape

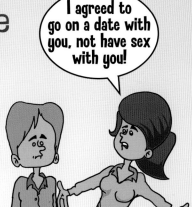

Rape is a type of sexual assault that can happen to males or females.

It involves:

- Penetration of the vulva, vagina, anus or mouth by a penis, body part (e.g. finger) or an object when a person did not consent or was not able to give consent.

Date rape happens when:

- Someone a person has just met or is going out with forces or manipulates them into having sex when they haven't given consent.

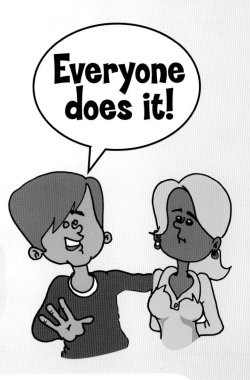

Regardless of the relationship, sexual contact without consent is against the law.

Rape and date rape are crimes

MYTHS ABOUT

There are many myths and untruths about sexual assault and sexual abuse. For example:

- MYTH: **'Women who wear sexy clothes are asking to be sexually assaulted.'**
False. No one asks or deserves to be sexually assaulted. It is a woman's choice to dress how she likes, for comfort or to look attractive.

- MYTH: **'It's not rape if the victim did not put up a fight.'**
False. One of the body's natural responses when threatened is to freeze. Regardless of whether the victim tried to defend themselves, it is still rape.

- MYTH: **'It's not rape if they are your partner.'**
False. Regardless of the relationship, sex without consent is rape.

- MYTH: **'Men cannot be sexually assaulted.'**
False. Both men and women can be sexually assaulted. In Australia, 2015, 1 in 20 men and 1 in 5 women over the age of 15 have been sexually assaulted.

SEXUAL ASSAULT

- MYTH: *'Most sexual assaults happen at night in dark quiet laneways.'*

False. Many sexual assaults happen in daytime and often in the home.

- MYTH: *'Most sexual assaults are committed by strangers.'*

False. 8 out of 10 victims are sexually assaulted by someone they know.

- MYTH: *'Some children let the abuse go on for a long time because they enjoy it.'*

False. Children often do not tell about sexual assault because the abuser may threaten or bribe them, or because they may feel ashamed or guilty. Sometimes they do not tell because they worry their family may not stay together.

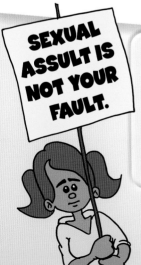

SEXUAL ASSULT IS NOT YOUR FAULT.

These myths try to excuse the behaviour of the wrongdoer (perpetrator) and suggest that they are not responsible for what they have done. This is not true! **People who commit sexual assault are responsible for their own actions.**

Support for people who have been sexually assaulted

If the sexual assault has just happened

If a young person has just been sexually assaulted, they could:

- Try to get to a safe place as soon as possible.
- Phone
  - Police on 000
  - Statewide Sexual Assault Helpline on 1800 010 120 or
  - Kids Help Line on 1800 551 800 (24 hour)
- Seek medical assistance as soon as possible, e.g.
  - Emergency Department at the local hospital,
  - local GP,
  - Family Planning Clinic or Sexual Health Clinic.

Medical examination can provide forensic information for legal purposes, testing for sexually transmitted infections, emergency contraception and referral for counselling and support.

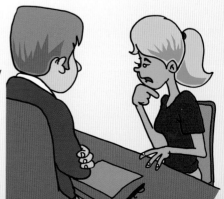

If the sexual assault or abuse occurred some time ago

Everyone has different feelings and reactions after sexual assault. Feelings may change from one day to the next or over a longer time. Sexual assault or sexual abuse may leave a person with feelings such as fear, shame, guilt, low self-esteem, depression or anxiety. Talking to someone about the experience, or about how they are coping with their life, can be helpful. This may assist them to have a more positive view of their future and increase the possibly that they will form satisfying future relationships.

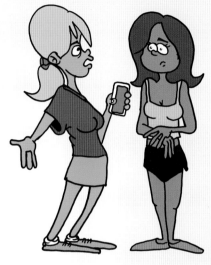

The local Sexual Assault Service or GP can arrange counselling.

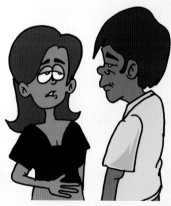

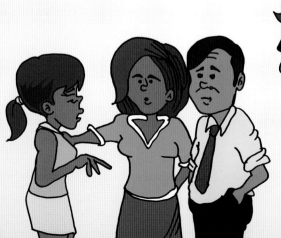

SEXTING

What is sexting?

When naked or intimate pictures are sent by SMS.

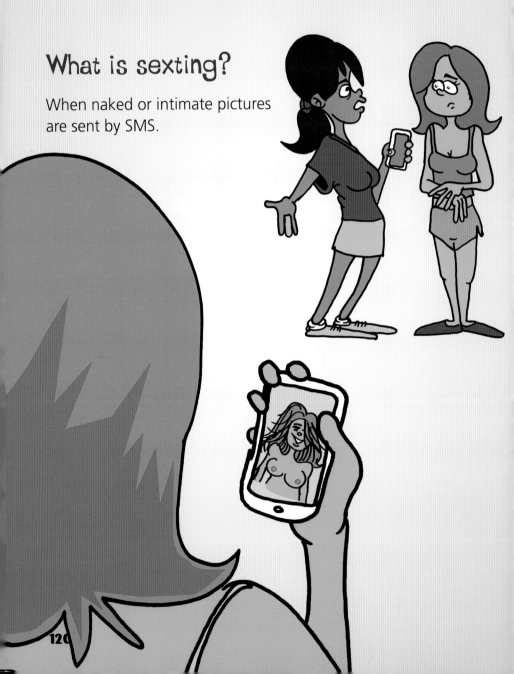

Why do people do this?

There can be many reasons. Maybe because someone they love has requested it. Maybe for a joke or just a bit of harmless fun. However, it is wise to consider what can happen later. The people who receive the images may save or forward them, or put them on a social networking site. This could lead to feelings of embarrassment, shame and humiliation.

What to do

Always take a minute or two to think about pictures that are being sent and who will receive them, even if it is someone close.

If pictures have already been sent and this causes regret, chat to a trusted adult. This could include the police.

If images are received, do not forward them. Delete them, and let the person know not to send any more.

If a person is being pressured to send images, they have the right to say 'NO!'. A person does not have to do anything that makes them feel uncomfortable, especially when they do not know where the pictures might end up. Images might even be viewed by classmates, parents, grandma or a future boss!

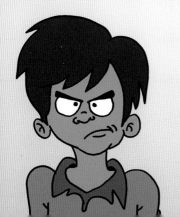 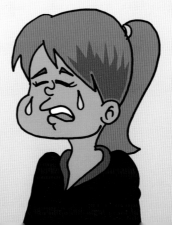

PORN

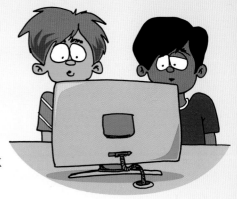

Porn (pornography) is:

'Printed and visual material that is intended to cause quick and intense sexual arousal'.

Porn is readily accessible online and many people watch it. Some young people are exposed to porn accidentally, while others search intentionally.

Online porn influences the attitude of many young people.

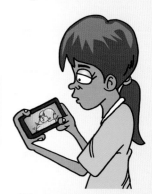

What they are learning from porn is misleading and confusing, and will not prepare them for healthy, respectful, consensual, safe sexual relationships.

Concerns about porn

1. Porn shows people being hurt

Porn usually shows women (and sometimes men) being hurt while they are involved in sexual acts. Some young people may see porn images that are hard to get out of their heads. They may have 'flash-backs' and nightmares about what they have seen.

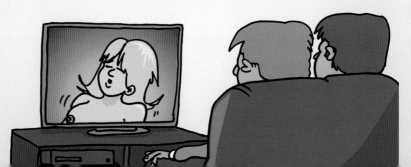

Porn does not show couples gaining consent, discussing contraception or what will give each other pleasure. In real life, people do not like to be forced or hurt.

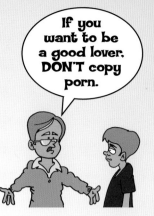

If you want to be a good lover, DON'T copy porn.

In real life, people want kind, gentle, considerate, loving partners.

2. Confusion about what is 'normal'

Males or females who watch porn might expect that they or their partner will look or behave like the people in porn movies. For example males will have a very large penis, and women will be slender, hairless, big breasted and beautiful.

Porn often shows women enjoying sexual acts that in real life usually do not give them any sexual pleasure. This is very confusing for young people who want a satisfying relationship. It is common for young men who watch porn to believe that their sexual partner will enjoy what is acted out in porn. *This is not the case!*

3. People may get 'hooked' on porn

Some people may find that they are unable to have a satisfying sex life without porn. People who watch porn often may watch it more and more, or watch increasingly aggressive material. Over time, they may develop strong feelings of guilt and shame, and become isolated from friends and family.

If anyone is worried about watching porn, images they have seen, or that they might be addicted to porn, they should talk to an adult they can trust, a counsellor or a doctor

Sex within a loving, respectful relationship is far more enjoyable and satisfying than the sex which is acted out in porn movies.

Emotional safety and wellbeing

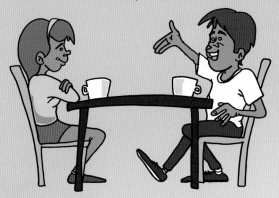

Partners who communicate, listen well and respect each other are building the foundations of a safe and enjoyable relationship. If relationships are not emotionally safe, people may feel used and hurt.

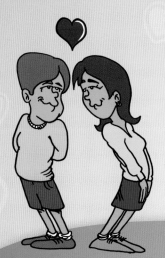

Thinking things through beforehand will help young people make the decision that is right for them. If they are still not sure about having sex, it may not be the right time or the right person.

The following '6Cs' sum up and say it all when young people are deciding whether to include sex in a relationship.

1 ♥ Consent
Both young people feel ready and consent to have sexual intercourse.

2 ♥ Communication
They are able to share their feelings, wants and needs.

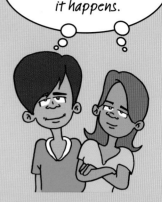

It's my decision who touches me and how and where it happens.

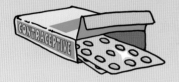

3 ♥ Condoms
They have condoms to prevent STIs.

4 ♥ Contraception
They have contraception to prevent pregnancy.

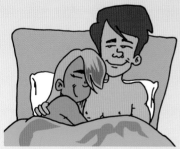

5 ♥ Comfort
They have a comfortable, safe and private place to have sex.

6 ♥ Care and consideration
They care about and are considerate of each other's feelings. They respect the privacy of the relationship.

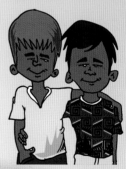

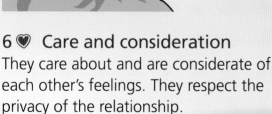

If the decision to have sex is made thoughtfully, is consistent with personal values and beliefs and people are emotionally ready, sex can be a wonderful part of a relationship.

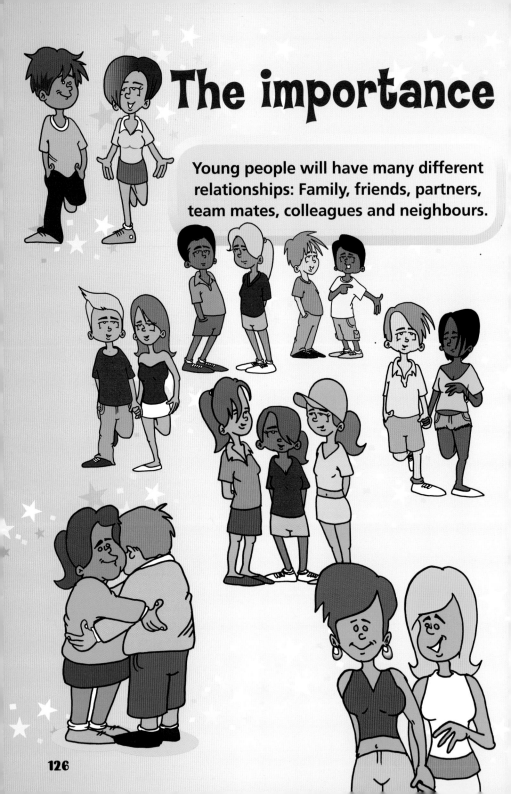

The importance

Young people will have many different relationships: Family, friends, partners, team mates, colleagues and neighbours.